DRINK THIS NOT THAT!

D0965417

THE
NO-DIET
WEIGHT LOSS
SOLUTION

Sip Your Way to a Flat Belly!
BY DAVID ZINCZENKO
WITH MATT GOULDING

RODALE

Eat This, Not That!, Drink This, Not That!, and Cook This, Not That!
are registered trademarks of Rodale Inc.

© 2010 by Rodale Inc.

All rights reserved. No part of this publication may be reproduced or transmitted in any form
or by any means, electronic or mechanical, including photocopying, recording, or any other information
storage and retrieval system, without the written permission of the publisher.

Rodale books may be purchased for business or promotional use or for special sales. For information,
please write to: Special Markets Department, Rodale Inc., 733 Third Avenue, New York, NY 10017.

Printed in the United States of America
Rodale Inc. makes every effort to use acid-free ♾, recycled paper ♺.

Book design by George Karabotsos

Photo direction by Tara Long

All interior photos by Mitch Mandel and Thomas MacDonald / Rodale Images
Food styling by Melissa Reiss

Cover photographs by Lucas Zarebinski
Food styling by Ed Gabriels; prop styling by Richie Owings; hand modeling by Ashly Covington

Illustrations on pages 110 to 119 by mckibillo

Library of Congress Cataloging-in-Publication Data is on file with the publisher

ISBN-13: 978-1-60529-539-8 paperback

Distributed to the trade by Macmillan

2   4   6   8   10   9   7   5   3   1   paperback

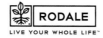

DEDICATION

To the more than 5 million Americans whose thirst
for knowledge about nutrition has led them to
the *Eat This, Not That!* and *Cook This, Not That!* series.
We'll keep fighting to make sure this well of
information never runs dry.

—Dave and Matt

Drink This, Not That!

ACKNOWLEDGMENTS

This book series is a collaborative effort in the truest sense, and *Drink This, Not That!* is no exception. Thanks to the dozens of exceptionally talented, passionate people who made this latest effort possible, especially:

To Maria Rodale and the Rodale family, who have worked tirelessly for four generations to educate America about the food we all eat.

To George Karabotsos and his dream team of designers, including Laura White, Mark Michaelson, Courtney Eltringham, Elizabeth Neal, and Rob Campos. You guys just keep getting better.

To Clint Carter, your knowledge and dedication have never been more critical and more appreciated than when applied to the world of liquids. Also, to Carolyn Kylstra, whose willingness to tackle any issue is more impressive than ever.

To Jeffery Lindemuth, whose remarkable wine and spirits expertise gives this book an incredible buzz. Thanks for being so damn good at what you do.

To Tara Long, our not-so-secret weapon—these books could not exist without you.

To Debbie McHugh, is there nothing you won't do to make sure we hit our deadlines? Thanks, as always, for your heroic efforts and extraordinary sacrifice.

To the immensely talented Rodale book team: Steve Perrine, Karen Rinaldi, Chris Krogermeier, Nancy N. Bailey, Sara Cox, Erin Williams, Mitch Mandel, Tom MacDonald, Troy Schnyder, Melissa Reiss, Nikki Weber, Staci Foley, Jennifer Giandomenico, Wendy Gable, Keith Biery, Liz Krenos, Brooke Myers, Sonya Maynard, Sean Sabo, and Caroline McCall. Every one of you plays a vital role in ensuring we deliver the highest-quality books to as many people as possible. Thank you.

And to our family, friends, and loved ones—cheers to you!

—Dave and Matt

Check out the other informative books in the EAT THIS, NOT THAT!® and COOK THIS, NOT THAT!™ series:

Eat This, Not That! (2007)	*Eat This, Not That! for Kids!* (2008)	*Eat This, Not That! Supermarket Survival Guide* (2009)	*Eat This, Not That! The Best (& Worst!) Foods in America!* (2009)	*Eat This, Not That! 2010* (2009)	*Eat This, Not That! Restaurant Survival Guide* (2009)	*Cook This, Not That! Kitchen Survival Guide* (2009)

CONTENTS

INTRODUCTION

It may be the most instantly gratifying pleasure known to man: That first cold, refreshing sip of your favorite beverage on a hot summer's day.

It might be a sweet, biting cola over ice, a cold beer straight from the fridge, or a glass of quick-mix lemonade. But when it slips past the lips, bounces over the tongue, and hits that dry spot in the back of your throat, bam! You're happy.

And when the weather turns cold, rainy, or sour? A beverage is still the fastest way to warm up the chill and turn your mood around: The bitter wake-up call of fresh-brewed coffee, the comforting sweetness of hot chocolate, the aromatic holiday cheer of a mulled cider. Whether it's time to celebrate (with a strawberry shake or a glass of champagne) or time to seek solace (with a comforting cup of tea or a misery-drowning martini), the right drink at the right time always seems to be the right answer.

What could possibly be wrong with that?

Well, here's what's wrong with that: While a drink may be the fastest way to quench a thirst or comfort a chill, it's also the fastest way to blow up a waistline. Here's a crazy statistic: More than 40 percent of Americans are on a diet at any given time. But while so many of us try to focus on watching

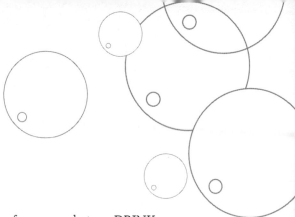

what we eat, the real way to lose weight is to focus on what we DRINK. Liquid calories now account for a whopping 21 percent of our daily calorie intake—more than 400 calories every single day, more than twice as much as we drank 30 years ago.

To give you a perspective on those numbers, imagine if you tossed two slices of Domino's sausage pizza into a blender, pressed "puree," and then guzzled it down. Presto, 450 calories. Now imagine doing that every single day for a year. Wow. Disgusting, right?

Yes, but behind those slightly sickening statistics is actually some terrific news. Because if you really want to lose weight—if you want to strip away fat (especially belly fat) and begin to sculpt a leaner, fitter body—you don't have to stop eating your favorite foods. In fact, you don't really have to watch what you eat at all. Just making some simple swaps in what you DRINK will shave pounds off your body at a remarkable pace. A recent study at Johns Hopkins University found that people who cut liquid calories from their diets lose more weight—and keep it off longer—than people who cut food calories. Simply cutting your drink calories in half—cutting back to what the average American drank just 30 years ago—could mean shaving off more than 23 pounds in just one year!

So, ready to hop on the wagon? Let's go!

America's Drinking Problem

On the African savannah, the watering hole is where all the action is. It's also where all the danger is. Every creature on Earth needs water, so if you are a crafty but lazy predator and want to lie in wait for dinner, the watering hole is the place to be. Lions lurk in the brush; crocodiles hover below the murky surface. Antelopes and zebras approach cautiously, needing a drink to survive, but worried they won't survive the drink.

Eons ago, humans faced the same dilemma as the antelope and the zebra. Jack and Jill went to fetch a pail of water, and—oh, snap!—Jack wound up as gator bait. Then we got hip: We created wells and aqueducts to carry water from the scary places it collected to the safe places where we needed it. From there, we could imbibe at our leisure: We could brew coffee, tea, or beer, or add herbs or fruits or sugar into our water to create new tastes, or cook up just about any beverage we could imagine, thanks to the miracles of modern plumbing. Later, after we invented cars and commerce, we could swing down to the drive-in or the soda shop for a Coke or a malt.

But then something happened. Over the past 50 years or so, we Americans have developed a severe drinking problem.

We stopped making our own iced teas and lemonades (recipe: water, lemon, sugar) and started buying them in bottles or mixes, with ingredients like "high-fructose corn syrup" and "ascorbic acid" on the labels. We stopped thinking of a soda as a treat—akin to an ice cream or a candy bar—and started seeing it as the equivalent of a glass of water, drinking two, three, four, or more a day. (The average American now drinks about a gallon of soda a week!) Then we stopped drinking water out of the tap and started demanding that

WORST WATER

While "Worst Water" may sound like an oxymoron, the devious minds in the bottled beverage industry have even found a way to besmirch the sterling reputation of the world's most essential compound. Sure, you may get a few extra vitamins, but ultimately, you're paying a premium price for gussied-up sugar water. Next time you buy a bottle of water, check the recipe: You want two parts hydrogen, one part oxygen, and very little else.

Sugar Equivalent:
2 Good Humor Chocolate Éclair Bars

Snapple
Agave Melon
Antioxidant Water
(1 bottle, 20 fl oz)
150 calories
0 g fat
33 g sugars

Drink This Instead!
Smartwater
0 calories
0 g sugars

20 WORST DRINKS IN AMERICA

America's supermarket aisles and drive-thru menus are awash in empty liquid calories. Survive the rising tide by eliminating these, the country's most damaging drinkables, from your beverage regiment.

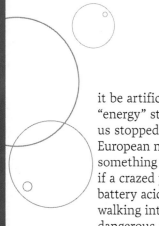

it be artificially flavored and put into bottles with the words "vitamin" or "energy" stamped on their labels. And, in just the last decade or so, many of us stopped brewing our own coffee and started buying things with vaguely European names, like "mocha latte," or swapped out coffee altogether for something called "energy drinks," which taste exactly like what would happen if a crazed pastry chef hijacked a truckload of Smarties and drove it into a battery acid factory. And the result of all this beverage evolution is that, today, walking into a convenience store or a beverage distributorship is almost as dangerous as sauntering down to that old African watering hole.

What happened? How did our drinking become so dangerous? Three things:

Beverages got cheaper to make. By replacing traditional sweeteners with artificial ones—either calorie-laden food derivatives like high-fructose corn syrup or calorie-free chemical experiments like aspartame or sucralose—companies like PepsiCo and Coca-Cola were able to produce billions of cans and bottles a year without needing to worry about the price of sugar. (By its own estimates, the Coca-Cola Company alone eats up 5 percent of all the sugar produced on planet Earth every year.)

Packages got cheaper to make. As little as 30 years ago—1980, to be exact—the average person drank most of his or her water out of the tap. Americans consumed just about 2½ gallons of bottled water annually. Today, that number is close to 30 gallons. That dramatic swing started with the 1973 patent of PET bottles (for polyethylene terephthalate), the plastic now used in the majority of soda and water bottles. (Eighty-five percent of all Coke products are now delivered in PET bottles.) With heavy, breakable, expensive-

WORST BOTTLED TEA

Leave it to SoBe to take an otherwise healthy bottle of tea and inject it with enough sugar to turn it into dessert. The Pepsi-owned company's flagship line, composed of 11 flavors with names like "Nirvana" and "Cranberry Grapefruit Elixir," is marketed to give consumers the impression that it can cleanse the body, mind, and spirit. Don't be fooled. Just like this bottle of green tea, all of these beverages are made with two primary ingredients: water and sugar.

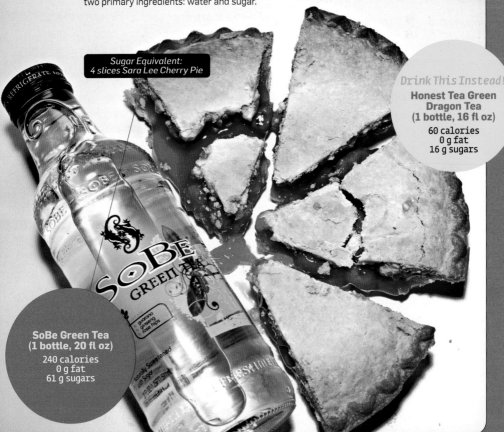

Sugar Equivalent:
4 slices Sara Lee Cherry Pie

Drink This Instead!
Honest Tea Green Dragon Tea (1 bottle, 16 fl oz)
60 calories
0 g fat
16 g sugars

SoBe Green Tea (1 bottle, 20 fl oz)
240 calories
0 g fat
61 g sugars

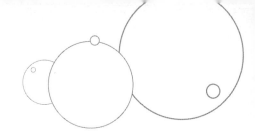

to-produce glass no longer necessary for their products, beverage manufacturers cut their costs dramatically. So it was easy to direct their money from manufacturing to marketing—and convince us that a bottle of Poland Spring was healthier than, say, tap water from Philadelphia.

Beverage marketers started getting "creative." Here are four pretty healthy-sounding words: Agave. Melon. Antioxidant. Water. Got them in your head? Good. Mix them up in a tall glass, over ice. Stir. Now take a sip. Can you taste the cool, refreshing splash of clean, crisp water and healing rain-forest fruits delivering their tropical bounty down your throat and into your cells? Yum. Good for you. Except if you're drinking something called Snapple Tropical Mango Antioxidant Water, in which case you're drinking 150 calories of pure sugar along with your H_2O. (Drinking just one of these concoctions a day in place of plain water will add more than 15 pounds to your body in the course of a year.) And those antioxidants? Two of them are fat-soluble vitamins A and E, which means that in a fat-free beverage like this, your body will have a hard time absorbing them. An hour or so after paying for them, you'll be flushing them good-bye.

As a result of all these developments, among the most basic functions of life, the second one we learn to do out of the womb (after we take our first breath), has become complicated and fraught with hazard. The cheapness of ingredients and packaging and the willingness of consumers to try new flavors not found in nature (go lick a mountain and tell me if it tastes like Mountain Dew) have given beverage manufacturers free license to manipulate our taste buds and try to find what researchers call our "bliss point"—the flavor point at which we get the greatest pleasure from sugar, fat, or salt. "Alone among the senses,

WORST ENERGY DRINK

None of the energy provided by these full-sugar drinks could ever justify the caloric load, but Rockstar's take is especially frightening. One can provides nearly as much sugar as half a box of Nilla Wafers. In fact, it has 60 more calories than the same amount of Red Bull and 80 more than a can of Monster. If you're going to guzzle, better choose one of the low-cal options. We like Monster; it offers all the caffeine and B vitamins with just enough sugar to cut through the funky extracts.

Sugar Equivalent:
6 Krispy Kreme Original Glazed Doughnuts

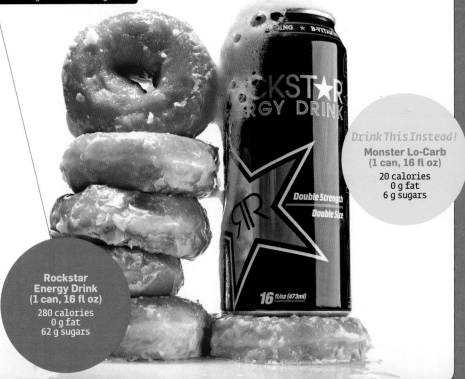

Drink This Instead!
**Monster Lo-Carb
(1 can, 16 fl oz)**
20 calories
0 g fat
6 g sugars

**Rockstar
Energy Drink
(1 can, 16 fl oz)**
280 calories
0 g fat
62 g sugars

taste is hardwired to brain cells that respond to pleasure," writes former FDA commissioner David Kessler, MD, in his book *The End of Overeating.* "It prompts the strongest emotional response."

So it's no wonder that beverage makers can get away with some of the monstrosities they're selling us as "refreshment." Consider some of the calorie equivalents you'll discover once you really start eyeing your drinks skeptically:

One Naked Protein Zone Juice smoothie

=

8 Fudgsicles

One Starbucks venti Peppermint White Chocolate Mocha

=

152 cups of black coffee

(or, in food equivalents, 26 cups of Orville Redenbacher's Natural Buttery Salt & Cracked Pepper Popcorn)

One Red Lobster Traditional Lobsterita

(there's something known as a "traditional" lobsterita? As opposed to those newfangled lobsteritas?)

=

2 Wendy's ¼ Pound Singles

And so today, you and I and the rest of America will drink about 21 percent of the total number of calories we're supposed to eat in an entire day. (And then we'll probably eat more total calories than we're supposed to eat, as well.)

Or: We can take the first step toward making effortless weightloss a reality. After all, if beverage manufacturers are going to make effortless weight gain a reality, don't you think it's time we fought back?

WORST BOTTLED COFFEE

With an unreasonable number of calorie landmines peppered across Starbucks' in-store menu, you'd think the company would want to use its grocery line to restore faith in its ability to provide caffeine without testing the limits of your belt buckle. Guess not. This drink has been on our radar for years, and we still haven't managed to find a bottled coffee with more sugar. Consider this—along with Starbucks' miniature Espresso and Cream Doubleshot—your worst option for a morning pickup.

Drink This Instead!

Illy Issimo Caffè
(1 can, 6.8 fl oz)

50 calories
0 g fat
11 g sugars

Starbucks Vanilla
Frappuccino
(1 bottle, 13.7 fl oz)

290 calories
4.5 g fat
(2.5 g saturated)
45 g sugars

Sugar Equivalent: 32 Nilla Wafers

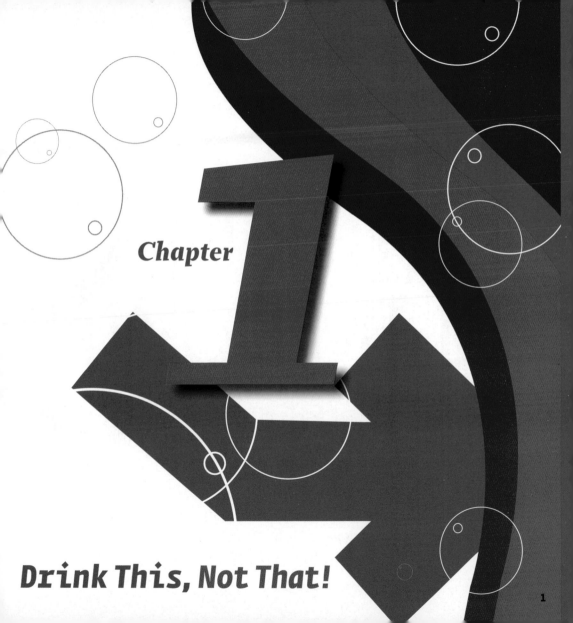

Chapter

1

Drink This, Not That!

DRINK UP SLIM DOWN

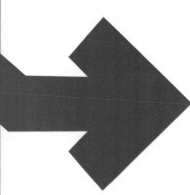

Imagine for a moment that you met a wizard, and he offered you a potion that would magically strip away pounds from your body, improve your overall health, lengthen your life, make you more attractive to the opposite sex, and keep you lean forever.

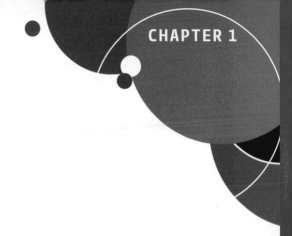

And imagine he told you that you could have a lifetime supply of said potion, for free. You'd probably have two questions:

Why the pointy hat?

And

What's the catch?

Well, imagine that I am that wizard. (Except with much better fashion sense. Pointy hats are soooo fifth century.) And my offer stands, with no catch at all: You can have all the magic weight-loss potion you want, for free, and start stripping away pounds— perhaps even several dozen pounds this year alone—without exercise, without dieting, without even visiting the set of *Nip/Tuck*.

What is this magical elixir? It's water.

Oh, come on! Really? Surely losing enormous amounts of weight isn't possible just by drinking water, is it? Don't I need any of that fancy fat-burning stuff they sell down at the local vitamin store?

No. In fact, the less you supplement your food and beverage intake, the more weight you'll lose (and the more money you'll save). In this chapter, we are going to walk you through a five-point plan for literally drinking away the pounds. And you're going to achieve your weight-loss goals without changing the way you eat, or even having to exercise. (Although once you start losing so much weight so fast, you're going to be inspired to eat better and exercise a little because you're going to be looking so incredibly good.) It's simply a matter of adjusting your choice of quaff.

It does sound too good to be true—until you start to look into the science. Then you'll see just how much of America's weight problem isn't an eating issue—it's a drinking issue.

Ready to take a ride with the wizard? Then start drinking up—and start slimming down!

Step 1 Swear Off the Soda and Iced Tea
(Annual Weight Loss: 20 Pounds!)

A lot of scientists, public health experts, statisticians, and other folks who always have pencil sharpeners at the ready have spent a lot of time trying to figure out what's caused America's obesity crisis.

Theories abound: One holds that we don't exercise enough because we spend most of our time working at our desks, driving around in our cars, or sinking into our sofas. Another states that it's our fast-food culture: We eat too much junk and not enough real food. And, most recently, many researchers have even theorized that our environment is playing a role, and

that everyday household chemicals are messing up our hormones and causing our bodies to store fat.

What are the chances that everybody is right? Well, actually, everybody *is* right, to a certain extent. We definitely eat too much junk, most of us don't get enough exercise, and we most certainly should be careful about exposing our sensitive endocrine systems to environmental pollutants (what experts are now calling "obesogens"). But by far the biggest contributor to our national weight problem is the fact that we drink too many calories. And the vast majority of those calories come to us from soda and other sweetened beverages.

Consider this: The National Health and Nutrition Examination Survey (NHNES), a government nutritional study conducted from 1999 to 2000, measured, among other things, where most of our calories come from. Researchers broke up America's food intake into 143 different categories and discovered, to their horror, that the category making up the largest percentage of our calorie intake—7.1 percent, to be exact—was not a food at all. It was soda. (Vegetables, on the other hand, accounted for only 6.5 percent of our intake. Chicken

WORST SODA

Wait . . . but aren't all sodas equally terrible? It's true they all earn 100 percent of their calories from sugar, but that doesn't mean there aren't still varying levels of atrocity. Despite the perception of healthfulness, fruity sodas tend to carry more sugar than their cola counterparts, and none make that more apparent than the tooth-achingly sweet Sunkist. But what seals the orange soda's fate on our list of worsts is its reliance on the artificial colors yellow 6 and red 40—two chemicals that may be linked to behavioral and concentration problems in children.

Sugar Equivalent:
6 Breyers Oreo Ice Cream Sandwiches

Drink This Instead!
Izze Sparkling Clementine
(1 bottle, 12 fl oz)
120 calories
0 g fat
27 g sugars

Sunkist
(1 bottle, 20 fl oz)
320 calories
0 g fat
84 g sugars

and fish together only added up to 5.7 percent.) To put that into perspective, if you were on a diet of 3,000 calories a day, and you cut 7 percent of your calories, you'd automatically drop down to 2,790, a difference that would save you 1.8 pounds per month. You could be 10 pounds lighter in 6 months by going cold-turkey today! (Oh, and by the way: You'll also be healthier, sexier, and richer, too. Don't believe me? Check out Chapter 3!)

Step 2 Drink 8 Cups of Ice Water Every Day
(Annual Weight Loss: 26 Pounds!)

Yes, the magic elixir really does have amazing powers. In one study, a group of 173 overweight women were put through diet and nutrition training using mainstream diet programs. Researchers then followed them for 10 months, with dietary and body composition being recorded up to 12 months after the classes. All women in the program lost weight, but those drinking more water lost more weight. Drinking more than 1 liter of water per day (nearly 4½ cups) was associated with an extra 5.07 pounds lost in 12 months.

And researchers from the University of Utah found that people who drink the most water have higher metabolisms. In a study, subjects drank 4, 8, or 12 cups of water each day. Those who drank at least 8 cups reported better concentration and higher energy levels, and tests showed that they were burning more calories than the 4-cups-a-day group.

Pretty cool, especially when you consider that almost 60 percent of your body—and most of your brain—is water. (In fact, a lot of both our hunger and our fatigue doesn't come from a lack of food or sleep, it comes from dehydration. More water = less hunger + more energy.)

While just drinking water will help you shed pounds, we're going to crank it up a notch (or three). Here's how:

Make it ice water. Add ice to that water, and you'll suddenly burn 64 more calories a day. The reason: Your body is running at 98.6 degrees, but the ice water is coming down your gullet at about 32. That means you need to use calories to cook that ice water up to body temperature so you can use it. More ice water means a higher metabolism, and more calories burned.

Drink the moment you wake up. The legendary Gracie family—the family that invented Brazilian jujitsu and, in

WORST BEER

Most beers carry fewer than 175 calories, but even your average extra-heady brew rarely eclipses 250. That makes Sierra's Bigfoot the undisputed beast of the beer jungle. Granted, the alcohol itself provides most of the calories, but it's the extra heft of carbohydrates that helps stuff nearly 2,000 calories into each six-pack. For comparison, Budweiser has 10.6 grams of carbs, Blue Moon has 13, and Guinness Draught has 10. Let's hope the appearance of this gut-inducing guzzler in your fridge is as rare as encounters with the fabled beast himself.

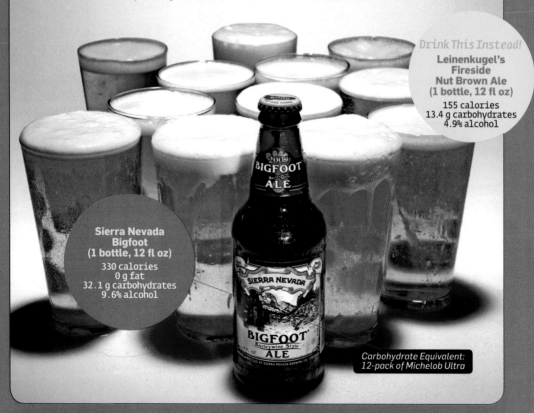

Drink This Instead!
Leinenkugel's Fireside Nut Brown Ale (1 bottle, 12 fl oz)
155 calories
13.4 g carbohydrates
4.9% alcohol

Sierra Nevada Bigfoot (1 bottle, 12 fl oz)
330 calories
0 g fat
32.1 g carbohydrates
9.6% alcohol

Carbohydrate Equivalent: 12-pack of Michelob Ultra

essence, Ultimate Fighting—lives by a code of always being ready to fight. (Bet they spend an awful lot of money replacing furniture . . .) And the first thing every Gracie does when he wakes up is to drink a big glass of water because being ready to fight means being properly hydrated. Now it turns out their tradition makes sense even for those of us who don't like getting punched in the face repeatedly. A study in the *Journal of the American Dietetic Association* found that drinking a glass of water before breakfast can cut daily food intake by 13 percent. So on top of the calories you're saving by swapping soda for H_2O, you're saving another 200 or so by staving off hunger! (That's another 21 pounds gone in a year!)

Drink before each meal. Researchers from Virginia Tech served 34 over-weight individuals breakfast on 2 separate days—once with a 16-ounce glass of water consumed 30 minutes before and once without. The average caloric intake on the day the group drank water before eating was 13 percent lower than on the day they went without the water.

(For more on our favorite beverage, check out the sidebar "Our Hero, H_2O" on page 12.)

Step 3 Enjoy One, Two or Even Three Yogurt-Based Smoothies a Day

(Annual Weight Loss: 10 Pounds!)

I love the sound of a cranking blender. But a combination of ice, dairy, and fruit does more than just make a teeth-rattling cacophony in your blender. It also helps strip pounds from your body.

There are three simple reasons why: Smoothies take little time to make (so you can quash your hunger pangs quickly); they're packed with nutrition (especially if you start with Greek yogurt and add berries, whey protein, and some flax); and their thickness takes up a lot of space in your stomach, crowding out the Doritos. In fact, researchers at Purdue University found that people stayed fuller longer when they drank thick drinks than when they drank thin ones, and a study at Penn State found that people who drank yogurt shakes that had been blended until they doubled in volume ate 96 fewer calories a day than those consuming thinner drinks.

And if that's not enough evidence for you, consider this: A University of Tennessee study found that men who

WORST KID'S DRINK

Don't let Tropicana's reputation for unadulterated OJ lead you to believe that the company is capable of doing no wrong. As a Pepsi subsidiary, it's inevitable that they'll occasionally delve into soda-like territory. The Twister line is just that: a drink with 10 percent juice and 90 percent sugar laced with a glut of artificial flavors and coloring. You could actually save 200 calories by choosing a can of Pepsi instead.

Sugar Equivalent:
Two 7-ounce canisters Reddi-wip

NATURALLY AND ARTIFICIALLY
Tropical Fruit
Fury FLAVORED

Tropicana
TW!STER

Drink This Instead!
Honest Kids Tropical Tango Punch
(1 pouch, 6.75 fl oz)
40 calories
0 g fat
10 g sugars

Tropicana Tropical Fruit Fury Twister
(1 bottle, 20 fl oz)
340 calories
0 g fat
60 g sugars

added three servings of yogurt a day to their diets lost 61 percent more body fat—and 81 percent more belly fat!—than men who didn't consume yogurt. The reason: Researchers think that calcium helps your body burn fat and helps limit the amount of new fat your body can make.

Step 4 Don't Drink Juice Drinks
(Annual Weight Loss: 19 Pounds!)

Imagine a world in which we called products what they really were: Hungry Man Dinners would be called Lonely Man Dinners. ESPN would be called the Fat Nerds Yap about Jocks Channel. And SunnyD would be called Obesi-D because there's nothing sunny about a drink marketed to kids that looks and tastes like juice, but is 95 percent water and corn syrup.

While even 100 percent juice has its problems (you'll read more about those in Chapter 5), juice drinks and their ilk are the worse offenders. One 16-ounce bottle of SunnyD Smooth packs a whopping 180 straight-up empty calories and 40 grams of sugar. If you drink one a day, cut it out. You'll lose 19 pounds in a year!

Step 5 Drink Coffee, Not Coffee Drinks
(Annual Weight Loss: 18 Pounds!)

Researchers studied coffee habits in New York and found that two-thirds of Starbucks' customers opted for blended coffee drinks over regular brewed coffee or tea. The average caloric impact of the blended drinks was 239 calories. The regular coffee or tea, by comparison, was only 63 calories after factoring in added cream and sugar. So even if you like your coffee sweet and light, you can strip away 176 calories every day, just by making this one swap.

Now, budding mathematicians among you may notice that all this adds up to a whopping 93 pounds lost in a single year. This is not good news if you weigh 125. (However, travel just got a lot cheaper because now you can mail yourself all over the world.)

Of course, unless you're currently engaging in all of the bad habits above, you probably don't have 93 pounds to lose. But this chapter illustrates how extraordinarily easy it is to shed extra weight—tons of weight—just by watching what we drink.

And that, my friends, is something worth raising a glass to.

WORST FUNCTIONAL BEVERAGE

Obviously Arizona took great pains in making sure this can came out looking like something you'd find in a pharmacy. But if your pharmacist ever tries to sell you this much sugar, he should have his license revoked. And if it's energy you're after, this isn't your best vehicle. Caffeine is the only compound in the bottle that's been proven to provide energy, and the amount found within is about what you'd get from a weak cup of coffee.

Sugar Equivalent:
6 Cinnamon Roll Pop-Tarts

Drink This Instead!

Glaceau Vitamin Water 10 Revitalize Green Tea (1 bottle, 20 fl oz)

25 calories
0 g fat
8 g sugars

Arizona Rx Energy (1 can, 23 fl oz)

345 calories
0 g fat
83 g sugars

Our Hero,
H$_2$O

Why you need more of the world's greatest beverage in your life

In his popular book *In Defense of Food*, Berkeley professor and author Michael Pollan summed up the overwhelming abundance of nutritional research, theories, and advice with seven simple words: Eat food. Not too much. Mostly plants.

We'd like to recalibrate his sagely advice for the liquid world with our own seven-word dictum. If you were to take away anything from this book, it should be this:

Drink water. Lots of it. Mostly tap.

Americans will spend more than $70 billion this year on bottled and packaged beverages produced by about 3,000 different companies, all in the name of quenching their collective thirst. And not even 20 percent of that will be spent on water. Maybe that's why we're drinking so little agua because we're filling our bellies instead with soda, sugary coffee drinks, and so-called functional beverages.

Just how little are we drinking?

According to a survey from the Cornel Medical Center, 75 percent of Americans are "chronically dehydrated." On top of that already troubling finding, a 7-year study conducted by the National Institutes of

WORST JUICE IMPOSTER

The twisted minds at the Arizona factory outdid themselves with this nefarious concoction, a can the size of a bazooka loaded with enough of the sweet stuff to blast your belly with 42 sugar cubes. The most disturbing part isn't that it masks itself as some sort of healthy juice product (after all, hundreds of products are guilty of the same crime), but that this behemoth serving size costs just $.99, making its contents some of the cheapest calories we've ever stumbled across.

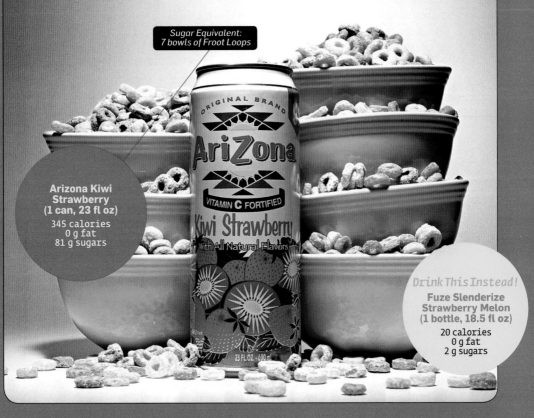

Sugar Equivalent:
7 bowls of Froot Loops

Arizona Kiwi Strawberry
(1 can, 23 fl oz)

345 calories
0 g fat
81 g sugars

Drink This Instead!
Fuze Slenderize
Strawberry Melon
(1 bottle, 18.5 fl oz)

20 calories
0 g fat
2 g sugars

Health, among others, found that Americans on average are consuming just over a liter of water a day—about half of what we should be taking in. In our opinion, this amounts to a national crisis. Not only does this have grave implications for most of our bodily functions, but reduced water intake has also been linked to fatigue, loss of concentration, and slower metabolisms. So it's not just our overall well-being, it's also our waistlines that are being affected by our apparent aversion to H_2O.

Here's what you need to do:

Purchase a water filter (a basic pitcher from Brita will run you about $20) and keep it constantly filled with plain old tap water. (Why tap? Read "The Truth About Bottled Water" on page 32 to find out.)

At work, keep a glass on your desk and drink from it constantly. (Add a straw—it helps you drink faster.) Make it a priority to drink water at every major transitional period throughout the day: when you wake up, as you leave the house, before and after each meal, when you call it a day at work, and before you go to bed.

What's that? Water's too boring for you? Then don't settle; use any of these zero-calorie tweaks to make your hydrogen-oxygen cocktail a little more interesting for your taste buds.

Add punch with produce.

Add slices of lemons, limes, or oranges to pitchers or glasses. Don't dig citrus? Both sliced apples and cucumbers add a nice subtle sweetness to a glass of water.

Turn your pitcher into an herb garden.

Fresh herbs add a variety of sweet, spicy, complex undertones to water. Add a big handful (our favorites are mint, basil, and tarragon) to a pitcher and use a wooden spoon to bash them up a bit— bruising the herbs will help release their flavor.

Harness your inner mixologist.

Treat water like a zero-calorie cocktail and see where your imagination and your mixing skills take you. Try spiking sparkling or still water with one of the dozens of flavors of sugar-free syrups—mango, raspberry, black cherry— offered from Torani.

WORST ESPRESSO DRINK

Hopefully this will dispel any lingering fragments of the "health halo" that still exists in coffee shops—that misguided belief that espresso-based beverages can't do much damage. In this 20-ounce cup, Starbucks manages to pack in more calories and saturated fat than two slices of deep-dish sausage and pepperoni pizza from Domino's. That makes it the equivalent of dinner and dessert disguised as a cup of coffee.

If you want a treat, look to Starbucks' supply of sugar-free syrups; if you want a caffeine buzz, stick to the regular joe, an Americano, or a cappuccino.

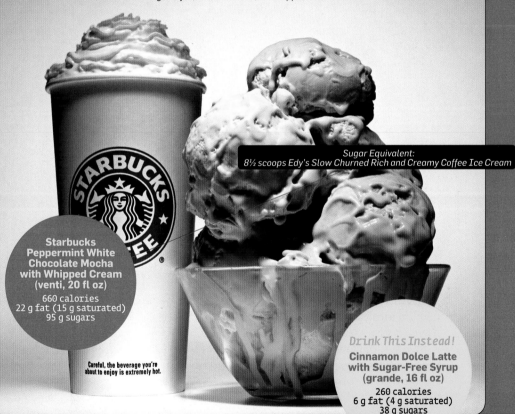

Sugar Equivalent:
8½ scoops Edy's Slow Churned Rich and Creamy Coffee Ice Cream

Starbucks Peppermint White Chocolate Mocha with Whipped Cream (venti, 20 fl oz)
660 calories
22 g fat (15 g saturated)
95 g sugars

Drink This Instead!
Cinnamon Dolce Latte with Sugar-Free Syrup (grande, 16 fl oz)
260 calories
6 g fat (4 g saturated)
38 g sugars

Careful, the beverage you're about to enjoy is extremely hot.

12 SECRETS THE BEVERAGE INDUSTRY DOESN'T WANT YOU TO KNOW

Baskin-Robbins doesn't want you to know that it takes a degree in food chemistry to engineer one of its "milk shakes." Think about the first milk shake you ever drank. Chances are it was chocolate or vanilla, blended in front of you by a young man wearing a paper hat and a toothy grin. And how many ingredients did he plop into that metal cup? Well, there was ice cream, milk, maybe a little syrup. Now contrast that with the Frankenshakes at Baskin-Robbins. Many of them can't be made with fewer than 30 ingredients. One, the Chocolate Chip Cookie

Dough Shake, requires a full 50—that's about 10 times what you would find in shakes at the ice cream parlors of yore.

So how did Baskin-Robbins inflate a five-ingredient indulgence into a 50-ingredient science-fair entry? Well, sugar, in its various forms, graces the ingredient list seven times. Partially hydrogenated oil, the source of trans fat, shows up three times. Then there's a smattering of flavoring agents such as artificial butter flavor, vanillin, and salt, and behind that comes the cabal of emulsifiers, thickeners,

WORST LEMONADE

There is no such thing as healthy lemonade, but Auntie's line of Lemonade Mixers takes the concept of hyper-sweetened juice and stretches it to dangerous new levels. See, sugar digests faster than good-for-you nutrients like protein and fiber, which means it's in your blood almost immediately after you swallow it. Drinking the 3 or 4 days' worth of added sugar found here jacks your blood sugar and results in strain to your kidneys, the creation of new fat molecules, and the desire to eat more. Ouch.

Auntie Anne's Wild Cherry Lemonade Mixer (32 fl oz)
470 calories
0 g fat
110 g sugars

Sugar Equivalent: 11 bowls of Cookie Crisp cereal

Drink This Instead!
Diet Lemonade (21 fl oz)
15 calories
0 g fat
0 g sugars

colors, and preservatives, industrial items such as guar gum, carrageenan, polysorbate 80, annatto color, potassium sorbate, sorbitan monostearate, and so forth. Basically it's what a milk shake would be if we ran out of real food and had to hand over the craft of culinary creation to chemists. Just as dismaying as the ingredient list is the nutritional breakdown: The large Cookie Dough Shake packs in 1,690 calories and 46 grams of saturated fat to go along with its 50 ingredients.

Ocean Spray doesn't want you to know that its line of cranberry juice blends contains more sugar than fruit. With enticing names such as Cran-Apple, Cran-Raspberry, and Cran-Pomegranate, Ocean Spray's bottles suggest that they're filled with nothing but the highest-quality juices. That's why you might be surprised to learn that many of them contain as little as 20 percent real juice. What's more, none of Ocean Spray's stable of hybrid "juices" earns fewer than 73 percent of its calories from added sugar, and most have sugar loads closer to 85 percent.

That amounts to about as much sugar as two scoops of ice cream stuffed into each 8-ounce cup of juice. The company tries to give it a natural spin by listing sugar on the ingredient statement as "cane or beet sugar," but as far as your body's concerned, it's no different from the table sugar used in the ice cream. You're better off thinking of these juices as noncarbonated soft drinks.

The dairy industry doesn't want you to know that the hormone rbST has been linked to cancer. If you've purchased milk anytime in the past decade, you've probably noticed that some jugs carry the claim: "from cows not treated with rbST." If you're among the more scrupulous consumers, you might have also noticed another, smaller claim: "No significant difference has been shown between milk derived from rbST-treated and non-rbST-treated cows." So what's with the rigmarole? Well, the first claim comes from legitimate fears about the carcinogenic effects of rbST, and the second comes from the successful efforts of lobbying on the behalf of its manufacturers.

See, rbST, recombinant bovine

WORST HOT CHOCOLATE

See that stack of Rice Krispie Treats? It's just three treats shy of two full boxes. Unless you were a contestant on *Fear Factor*—and there was a sizeable monetary prize on the line—you'd never even consider noshing down that much sugar at once. But here's what's interesting: While that stack is the sugar counterpart to this atrocity from Starbucks, it still has 40 percent less saturated fat. Makes us wonder what's going on in the hot chocolate. Stick to beverages with single-flavor profiles instead of pile-on recipes like this and you'll fare better every time.

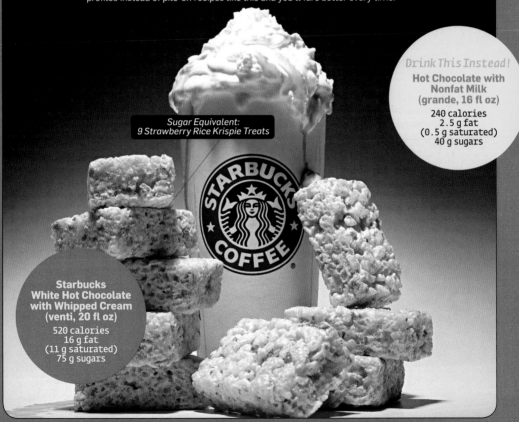

Sugar Equivalent:
9 Strawberry Rice Krispie Treats

Drink This Instead!

Hot Chocolate with Nonfat Milk (grande, 16 fl oz)

240 calories
2.5 g fat
(0.5 g saturated)
40 g sugars

Starbucks White Hot Chocolate with Whipped Cream (venti, 20 fl oz)

520 calories
16 g fat
(11 g saturated)
75 g sugars

somatotropin (also known as rBGH, recombinant bovine growth hormone), is a hormone given to cows to increase their milk output by 10 to 25 percent. It was developed by biotech monolith Monsanto, and after an unsuccessful attempt to convince consumers of its safety, it was sold to Elanco, a company that specializes in agricultural pharmaceuticals. Monsanto, for its part, fought hard to prevent dairy farmers from telling consumers whether their cows were treated with rbST. The dairy farmers fought back, and the result was the pairing of seemingly contradictory statements that now appear on the packaging of many milk cartons. The concern with rbST is that it produces milk with higher-than-normal levels of the insulin-like growth factor IGF-1. A series of studies at the Channing Laboratory in Boston showed that high levels of IGF-1 increased the risk of several cancers, including breast, prostate, and colorectal. In the study, those with the highest levels of the hormone were four times as likely to develop cancer. True, other studies contradict the findings, but until the issue is resolved, we recommend playing it safe. Especially when so many big players—Starbucks, Kroger, and Wal-Mart among them—have agreed to sell only hormone-free milk.

The diet soda industry doesn't want you to know that artificial sweeteners can make you fat. Let's be honest: People don't drink diet soda and truly believe they're doing their bodies any favors. Sure it's a step up from regular soda, but for every can of diet you drink, that's a cup of water or tea—genuinely healthy beverages—that you skipped over. But here's where's things get thorny: Although it's essentially calorie free, diet soda can drive your appetite and push you to overconsume calories.

Researchers at the University of Texas Health Science Center discovered this by collecting data on 622 people. Over a span of 8 years, every can of diet soda consumed on a daily basis amounted to a 41 percent jump in the risk of obesity. The researchers were quick to note that this probably doesn't represent a direct cause-and-effect relationship, but it does underscore the

WORST FROZEN COFFEE DRINK

Coffee-dessert hybrids are among the worst breed of beverages. This one delivers 1 gram of fat and 4.6 grams of sugar in every ounce, making even Starbucks' over-the-top line of Frappuccinos look like decent options. Maybe that's why DQ decided to give it a name that alludes to the animal it promises to turn you into. If you can bring yourself to skip DQ and head to a coffee shop instead, order a large iced latte with a couple shots of flavored syrup and save some 600 calories. But if you're stuck where you are, you're better off pairing a small treat with a regular cup of joe.

Dairy Queen Caramel MooLatte (24 fl oz)

870 calories
24 g fat
(19 g saturated, 1 g trans)
112 g sugars

Drink This Instead!

Small Chocolate Ice Cream Cone with a Medium Cup of Coffee

240 calories
7 g fat (5 g saturated)
25 g sugars

*Sugar Equivalent:
12 Dunkin' Donuts Bavarian Kreme Doughnuts*

confusion surrounding artificially sweetened beverages. Especially when considered alongside another study from Purdue: Researchers there fed saccharin to a group of rats and discovered that, compared with those eating sugar-sweetened foods, the saccharin rats gained more weight. One theory put forth by researchers is that giving the body a rush of sugar with no calories might push it to actively seek out sources of energy. And how does your body do that? By switching your appetite into overdrive.

The cocktail industry doesn't want you to know that high-fructose corn syrup is the primary ingredient in your libation. Tom Collins. Whiskey sour. Piña colada. What do they have in common? A massive load of sweetness waiting to highjack your blood sugar and send your body into fat-storage overdrive. Sure, the names allude to exotic fruits and high-society sophistication, but don't be fooled. From Manhattan to Margaritaville, your favorite cocktail mixer is probably saddled with twice as much sugar as your favorite soda. Most mixers follow the same basic recipe: water, high-fructose corn syrup, and a laundry list of thickeners, preservatives, and artificial flavors and colors. Down a few of those in an evening and you might as well have just polished off a bathtub full of Skittles, especially when you factor in the caloric impact of the booze. Want a mixer that's not pure garbage? Make it a Bloody Mary; it's almost always made from real pureed tomatoes. Look for the one with the most real juice and the lowest level of sodium. Or better yet—make yours with Spicy V8. It's 100 percent juice and has less sodium than most mixers.

7Up doesn't want you to know that it takes a centrifuge to produce their "all natural" soda. This might be the most flagrant abuse of the term "natural" we've seen. Even if you can overlook the fact that a 20-ounce bottle of 7Up has nearly as much sugar as five Breyers Oreo Ice Cream Sandwiches, that still leaves the issue of corn-derived sweeteners, which are about as "natural" as Mickey Rourke's nose.

To obtain the high-fructose

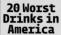

WORST MARGARITA

Drink This Instead!

Red Lobster Classic Margarita on the Rocks

250 calories
0 g fat
22 g carbohydrates

Traditional Red Lobster Lobsterita (24 fl oz)

890 calories
0 g fat
183 g carbohydrates

Carbohydrate Equivalent: 7 Almond Joy candy bars

Of all the egregious beverages we've analyzed, the Lobsterita surprised us the most. The nation's biggest fish purveyor is one of the few big players in the restaurant biz to provide its customers with a wide selection of truly healthy food options. We would hope they'd do the same with the beverages, but obviously not. Drink one of these every Friday night and you'll put on more than a pound of flab each month. Downgrade to a regular margarita on the rocks and pocket the remaining 640 calories.

corn syrup that spikes this bottle, processors must ship the corn to a facility that can crush it into a slurry of fiber, protein, and starch. A soaking process helps separate out the starch and the rest is stuffed into a centrifuge, a motorized, rotating piece of machinery (a perfect symbol of the unflagging ingenuity of the industrial food complex) to spin out the germ. That starch is blended with enzymes that convert it into dextrose, and then blended again with more enzymes to convert it into fructose. Finally, the glucose and fructose are stirred together to create a substance that has a flavor similar to table sugar. The process begs the question: If that's not natural, then what is?

7Up isn't the only company guilty of exploiting misunderstood terms to sling soda. Pepsi, Mountain Dew, and Snapple have all recently released versions of their popular beverages extolling the replacement of high-fructose corn syrup with regular cane sugar. Problem is, there's no proof cane sugar is any better for you; all you have is another can or bottle loaded with hundreds of empty calories. Don't be fooled.

The coffee industry doesn't want you to know that the average latte is worse than a double-scoop ice cream cone. Forget the 24-hour news cycle; ours is a 24-hour dessert culture. From lackluster smoothies and bran muffins at breakfast to chicken teriyaki bowls for dinner, we're unwittingly consuming sweets at every hour of the day.

And no source of sugar is more stealth than the caffeine kicks dished out at coffee shops across America. Even an unflavored 16-ounce latte has close to 200 calories, and for the average person that represents nearly 10 percent of your daily energy requirements. And once you start tagging on the extra embellishments, you can quickly find your way into the land of low-swinging bellies. Starbucks alone sells about two dozen drinks with more than 500 calories apiece. (And that's not even counting the absurdly indulgent and overwrought Frappuccinos.) Drink something like that once a day and you're facing at least an extra 50 pounds of flab each year! And what's worse, Starbucks isn't alone. It seems every coffee shop in the country is locked in an arms race for bigger, more

WORST FLOAT

Done right, an ice cream float can be a decent route to indulgence. Go to A&W and you'll land a medium for fewer than 400 calories. Order it with diet soda and you've dropped below 200 calories. So why can't Baskin-Robbins make even a small float with fewer than 470 calories? Because apparently the chain approaches the art of beverage-crafting as a challenge to squeeze in as much fat and sugar as possible. Whatever you order, plan on splitting it with a friend.

Baskin-Robbins Ice Cream Soda (vanilla ice cream and cola) (large, 28.6 fl oz)

960 calories
40 g fat
(25 g saturated,
1.5 g trans)
136 g sugars

*Sugar Equivalent:
9.7 Fudgsicle fudge bars*

Drink This Instead!

Ice Cream Float (vanilla ice cream and root beer) (small, 16.9 fl oz)

470 calories
20 g fat
(13 g saturated,
0.5 g trans)
68 g sugars

25

indulgent drinks. If you need an occasional fix for your sweet tooth, make it somewhere that isn't part of your daily routine. A couple scoops of regular coffee ice cream at Ben and Jerry's—one of the lighter ice creams on the menu—will cost you fewer than 400 calories. And when it comes to your caffeine fix, find it in regular coffee or unflavored espresso-and-milk drinks.

Glacéau doesn't want you to know that a bottle of Vitaminwater has more sugar than a Snickers bar. And yet, through ingenious marketing, they've managed to pass off their product as good for you! As if the 32.5 grams of sugar they stuff into each bottle—8 teaspoons' worth—was somehow going to improve your health!

Okay, let's be fair. What Glacéau really wants you to think is that the sugar is negligible (it isn't), and that the flurry of vitamins it drizzles into its bottles will improve your well-being (that's up for debate). See, the crutch of every bottle of Vitaminwater is a host of B vitamins. Everything that goes in after that—zinc, chromium, vitamins A, C, or E, etc.—hinges on whether

said beverage is trying to provide Focus, Sync, Balance, or any number of elusive and unsubstantiated health claims. The problem is this scant collection of nutrients isn't worth the stiff sugar tariff that Vitaminwater charges. If your diet is even remotely close to healthy, then you're probably already getting what you need. But if you're still concerned about getting all your nutrients, take a daily multivitamin, washed down with a cool, refreshing glass of zero-calorie water.

The beer and soda industries don't want you to know that aluminum cans are lined with a toxic plastic. You might have already heard of something called bisphenol A, otherwise known simply as BPA. It's a chemical found in plastics, and a series of studies have identified it as a threat to your health. At the University of Cincinnati, for instance, researchers found that low doses of BPA suppress a hormone that protects against diabetes and obesity in human tissue. Another study at the Yale School of Medicine discovered that BPA disrupts brain function and leads to mood disorders in monkeys. Add

WORST FROZEN FRUIT DRINK

Imagine taking a regular can of soda, pouring in 18 extra teaspoons of sugar, and then swirling in half a cup of heavy cream. Nutritionally speaking, that's exactly what this is, which is how it manages to marry nearly 2 days' worth of saturated fat with enough sugar to leave you with a serious sucrose hangover. Do your heart a favor and avoid any of Krispy Kreme's "Kremey" beverages. The basic Chillers aren't the safest of sippables either, but they'll save you up to 880 calories.

**Krispy Kreme
Lemon Sherbet Chiller
(20 fl oz)**

980 calories
40 g fat
(36 g saturated)
115 g sugars

*Sugar Equivalent:
16 medium-size chocolate eclairs*

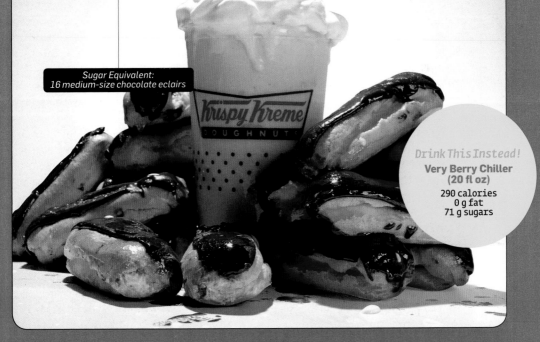

Drink This Instead!
**Very Berry Chiller
(20 fl oz)**

290 calories
0 g fat
71 g sugars

that to the growing pile of evidence that show it to lower sperm counts, up your risk of heart disease, and increase the risk of breast, prostate, and testicular cancers, and you have a pretty good reason for keeping it out of your diet.

Unfortunately that's easier said than done. Even if you've already replaced your plastic food containers with glass, you're still susceptible to a BPA bludgeoning from aluminum cans. Aluminum is highly reactive, so canners use a BPA-loaded epoxy lining to keep their contents safe. Several US jurisdictions have banned BPA from being used in baby bottles, and the USDA is evaluating its safety in other products. But don't expect major improvements anytime soon—the beverage industry is reluctant to part with its cheap fix. In 2009, the *Washington Post* uncovered internal documents from Coca-Cola that outlined a public-relations strategy for trying to persuade consumers that BPA was safe. In it, the soda moguls discussed the possibility of using fear tactics and targeting young mothers who make the most household purchasing decisions. Pretty scary stuff.

Smoothie King doesn't want you to know that two-thirds of the smoothies on its menu come spiked with sugar. Here's the rule of smoothies: Once sugar has been added to the cup, it can no longer be considered a smoothie. And yet, of the 91 blends on Smoothie King's menu, only 29 come without a lacing of sugar. Six of those are on the kids' menu, which really leaves you only 22 sans-sugar smoothies to choose from. Smoothie King justifies the affront by using only honey and turbinado sugar. We applaud the effort, but ultimately both sweeteners spike your blood sugar just as severely as the table sugar used to make cookies and candy.

Want to avoid the problem? Order your smoothie "skinny." At Smoothie King, that's code for "please give me a real smoothie instead of candied fruit." They'll happily give the skinny treatment to any smoothie you order, and for most 20-ounce flavors, that will save you about a hundred calories. In the most extreme cases, ordering skinny will slice 400 calories from a 40-ounce cup. That savings amounts to more calories than two steak soft tacos at Taco Bell.

WORST FROZEN MOCHA

A frozen mocha will never be a stellar option, but we've still never come across anything that competes with this cookie-coffee-milkshake hybrid from Così. Essentially it's a mocha Blizzard made with Oreo cookies and topped with whipped cream and an oversize Oreo. The result is a beverage with more calories than two Big Macs and more sugar than any other drink in America.

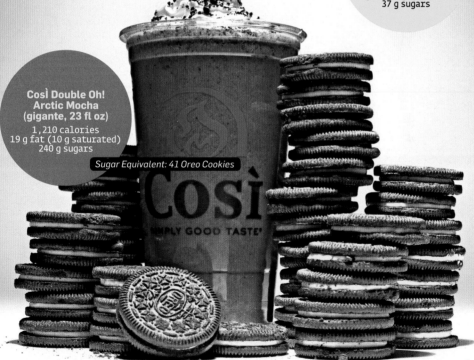

Così Double Oh! Arctic Mocha (gigante, 23 fl oz)

1,210 calories
19 g fat (10 g saturated)
240 g sugars

Sugar Equivalent: 41 Oreo Cookies

Drink This Instead!

Chocolate Covered Strawberry Smoothie (12 oz)

316 calories
12 g fat (8 g saturated)
37 g sugars

Juice companies don't want you to know what goes into 100 percent juice. Thanks to lax FDA regulations, industrial juicers have more than a little wiggle room when it comes to labeling their bottles. One loophole they love to exploit is the one that allows the claim "100 percent juice" to be used out of context with the other claims on the label, which is how they slap expensive-sounding names onto cheap juice blends. What these juicers know is that some juices—most notably apple, grape, and pear—are cheap, abundant, and loaded with sugar, so they look to these to stretch and sweeten more nutritious and expensive juices. You might think your bottle contains 100 percent blueberry or pomegranate, but really it's just as likely to be a blend of inexpensive sucrose-loaded fillers tinged with a mere splash of what you really want.

Instead of rewriting the regulation that allows this sort of fallacious language, the FDA sends out warning letters. Last year it chastised Nestlé for sticking bogus 100 percent juice claims on its grape- and orange/tangerine-flavored Juicy Juice products. That's little consolation for you, though. Juicy Juice is just one of dozens of inauthentic products in the juice aisle. We hope the government will start doing what's right for the consumer and start making these companies accountable.

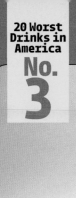

WORST DRIVE-THRU SHAKE

Drink This Instead!

**Hot Fudge Sundae
(small, 6.3 oz)**

330 calories
10 g fat (7 g saturated)
48 g sugars

**McDonald's
Triple Thick
Chocolate Shake
(large, 32 fl oz)**

1,160 calories
27 g fat
(16 g saturated,
2 g trans)
168 g sugars

*Sugar Equivalent:
13 McDonald's Baked Hot Apple Pies*

There are very few milk shakes in America worthy of your hard-earned calories, but few will punish you as thoroughly as this Mickey D's drive-thru disaster. Not only does it have more than half your day's caloric and saturated fat allotment and more sugar than you'd find in Willy Wonka's candy lab, but Ronald even finds a way to sneak in a full day of cholesterol-spiking trans fat. The scariest part about this drink is that it's most likely America's most popular milk shake.

The Truth About Bottled Water

Imagine you've just been given a choice: You have to drink from one of two containers. One container is a cup from your own kitchen, and it contains a product that has passed strict state, federal, and local guidelines for cleanliness and quality. Oh, and it's free. The second container comes from a manufacturing plant somewhere, and its contents—while seemingly identical to your first choice—have not been subjected to the same strict national and local standards.

It costs approximately four times more than gasoline. These products both look and taste nearly identical.

WHICH DO YOU CHOOSE?

If you chose beverage A, congratulations: You just saved yourself a whole lot of money and perhaps even contaminants, too. But if you picked beverage B, then you'll be spending hundreds of unnecessary dollars on bottled water this year. Sure, bottled water is convenient, trendy, and may well be just as pure

as what comes out of your tap. But it's hardly a smart investment for your pocketbook, your body, or our planet. We decided to take a closer look at what's behind the pristine images and elegant-sounding names printed on those bottles.

You may actually be drinking tap water.
Case in point: Dasani, a Coca-Cola product. Despite its exotic-sounding name, Dasani is simply purified tap water that's had minerals added back in. For

example, if your Dasani water was bottled at the Coca-Cola Bottling Company in Philadelphia, you're drinking Philly tap water. But it's not the only brand of water that relies on city pipes to provide its product. About 40 percent of all bottled water is taken from municipal water sources, including Pepsi's Aquafina.

Bottled water isn't always pure.
Scan the labels of the leading brands and you see variations on the words "pure" and "natural"

WORST SMOOTHIE

If Smoothie King wants someone to blame for landing this high on our worst beverages roundup (and truth be told, its entire menu is riddled with contenders), the chain should point the smoothie straw at whichever executive came up with the cup-sizing structure. Sending someone out the door with a 40-ounce cup should be a criminal offense. Who really needs a third of a gallon of sweetened peanut butter blended with grape juice, milk, and bananas? Sugar-and fat-loaded smoothies like this should be served from 12-ounce cups, not mini kegs.

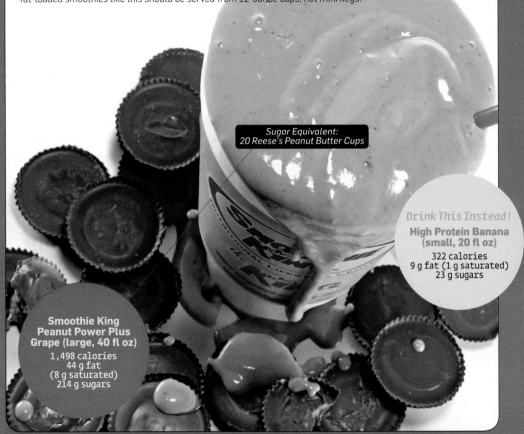

Sugar Equivalent:
20 Reese's Peanut Butter Cups

Drink This Instead!
High Protein Banana (small, 20 fl oz)
322 calories
9 g fat (1 g saturated)
23 g sugars

Smoothie King Peanut Power Plus Grape (large, 40 fl oz)
1,498 calories
44 g fat
(8 g saturated)
214 g sugars

and "pristine" over and over again. And when a Cornell University marketing class studied consumer perceptions of bottled water, they found that people thought it was cleaner, with less bacteria. But that may not actually be true. For example, in a 4-year review that included the testing of 1,000 bottles of water, the Natural Resources Defense Council—one the country's most ardent environmental crusaders—found that "about one-third of the brands we tested contained, in at least one sample, chemical contaminants at levels above strict state health limits."

Our country's high demand for oil isn't just because of long commutes.

Most water bottles are composed of a plastic called polyethylene terepthalate (PET). Now, to make PET, you need crude oil. Specifically, 17 million barrels of oil are used in the production of PET water bottles ever year, estimate University of Louisville scientists. No wonder the per-ounce cost of bottled water rivals that of gasoline. What's more, 73 percent of 36 billion PET water bottles sold annually are tossed in the trash instead of being recycled, according to data from the Container Recycling Institute.

That's a lot of waste—waste that will outlive you, your children, and your children's children. You see, PET bottles take 100 to 1,000 years to degrade. Which begs the question: If our current rate of consumption continues, where will we put all of this discarded plastic?

It's not clear where the plastic container ends and the drink begins.

Turns out that, when certain plastics are heated at a high temperature, chemicals from the plastics may leach into a container's contents. So there's been a flurry of speculation recently as to

whether the amounts of these chemicals are actually harmful, and whether this is even a concern when it comes to water bottles—which aren't likely to be placed in boiling water or even a microwave. While the jury is still out on realistic health ramifications, it seems that, yes, small amounts of chemicals from PET water bottles such as antimony—a semi-metal that's thought to be toxic in large doses—can accumulate the longer bottled water is stored in a hot environment. Which, of course, is probably a good reason to avoid storing bottled water in your garage for six months—or, better yet, to just reach for filtered tap instead.

WORST BEVERAGE IN AMERICA

In terms of saturated fat, drinking this Cold Stone catastrophe is like slurping up 68 strips of bacon. Health experts recommend capping your saturated fat intake at about 20 grams per day, yet this beverage packs more than three times that into a cup the size of a Chipotle burrito. But here's what's worse: No regular shake at Cold Stone, no matter what the size, has fewer than 1,000 calories. If you must drink your ice cream, make it one of the creamery's "Sinless" options. Otherwise you'd better plan on buying some bigger pants on the way home.

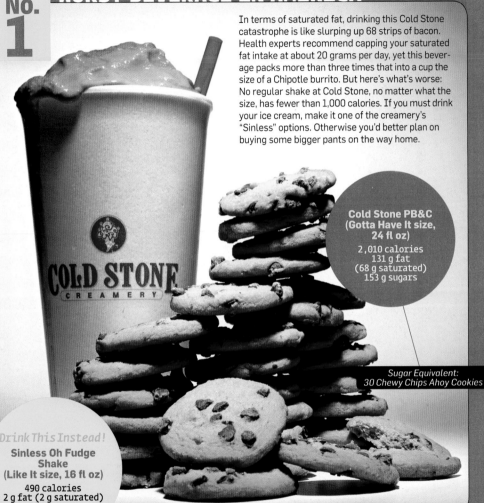

COLD STONE CREAMERY

**Cold Stone PB&C
(Gotta Have It size,
24 fl oz)**

2,010 calories
131 g fat
(68 g saturated)
153 g sugars

*Sugar Equivalent:
30 Chewy Chips Ahoy Cookies*

Drink This Instead!
**Sinless Oh Fudge Shake
(Like It size, 16 fl oz)**

490 calories
2 g fat (2 g saturated)
44 g sugars

Chapter

2

Drink This, Not That!

AT YOUR FAVORITE RESTAURANTS

Ever go to a carnival or a state fair and play one of those "games of skill and luck" that line the midway? You know, where you pay 2 bucks to toss a dart at a balloon or a softball through a clown's mouth and "everyone's a winner?"

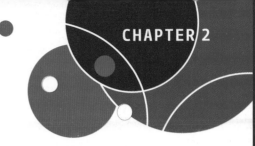
Did you ever wonder how it was possible that the barkers could give away so many prizes and still make a profit? It's simple. All the prizes are cheap, useless crap. The stuffed animals and toy critters are stitched together with inexpensive materials and designed to give the "winner" a couple of hours of enjoyment before being stuffed somewhere to idle uselessly, taking up space.

What does this have to do with your health? Plenty. The next time you walk into a chain restaurant and see that they're offering "bottomless" refills on soft drinks, keep that carnival barker in mind. Because what you're getting, in most cases, is something made of cheap materials, designed to give you brief moments of pleasure before being stuffed away—mostly in your fat cells—forever more.

As much as we might demonize Frisbee-size burgers and indecently stuffed pizzas that populate America's menus, in many ways what makes or breaks a meal is the beverage we wash

it down with. And just because those 44-ounce cups and endless refills of soda cost restaurant owners next to nothing doesn't mean they don't cost YOU quite a bit.

Nowhere are profit margins higher in the restaurant industry than with drinks. So cheap is the cost of soda that McDonald's is currently mulling over a plan to sell all drink sizes for a buck, which will inevitably spike demand (and profits) precipitously. So we're set up for failure, of both the financial and caloric nature.

The key to eating smart in a restaurant, then, is drinking smart in a restaurant. And that's what this chapter is all about: learning to ignore the carnival barkers.

10 Drinks Everyone Should Know How to Make

There's no better way to save precious dollars and even more precious calories than by learning to create your favorite beverages at home.

Smoothie

Power Smoothie

- 1 banana
- ½ cup milk
- ½ cup Greek-style yogurt
- ¼ cup orange juice
- ½ Tbsp peanut butter
- 1 Tbsp vanilla- or chocolate-flavored protein powder
- 1 Tbsp fiber powder (often sold as psyllium husk)
- 1 Tbsp flaxseed

The healthy reputation of the smoothie is one that is too often exploited by major drink purveyors, who use its good name to sling beverages that by any other definition should be labeled milk shakes. In a perfect world, smoothies should be long on fruit, fiber, and protein and short on sugar and unnecessary fat, traits that this Power Smoothie encapsulates perfectly. Its onslaught of vital nutrients— protein from the peanut butter and the powder; fiber from the fruit and the powder; omega-3s from the flaxseed—will not only help fill your stomach and charge your metabolism, but it will ensure peak performance all morning long.

How to Make It:
Place all the ingredients in a blender and blend until smooth and uniform.

Per serving:
350 calories
12 g fat
30 g sugars

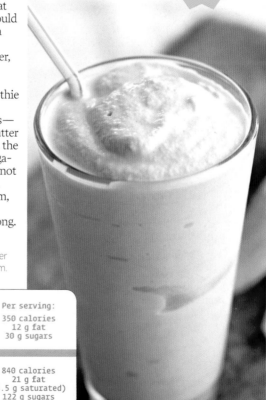

Not That!

Jamba Juice Peanut Butter Moo'd
(24 fl oz)

840 calories
21 g fat
(4.5 g saturated)
122 g sugars

Drink This!
Bloody Mary

Between the lycopene-rich tomato juice and the bevy of nutritient-packed garnishes, a strong case can be made that the Bloody Mary is the world's healthiest cocktail. The bloody is so solid that it's hard even for restaurants to screw up, except when they charge you $9 for a glass that contains 1,200 milligrams of sodium.

The Ultimate Bloody Mary

6 oz low-sodium V8

1½ oz vodka

3 to 4 dashes Worcestershire sauce

1 tsp horseradish (freshly grated is best, but the bottled stuff works in a pinch)

Tabasco to taste

Juice of ¼ lemon

Pinch of celery salt

A few grinds of freshly cracked pepper

Garnish: Fresh celery stick, olives, pickled vegetables like cocktail onions, green beans, and/or brussels sprouts

How to Make It:

Combine the V8, vodka, Worcestershire, horseradish, Tabasco, lemon juice, and celery salt in a pint glass. Use a spoon to stir vigorously. Fill the glass with ice and top with fresh cracked pepper. Garnish with a celery stick and as many different pickled vegetables as you can get your hands on.

Mix It Up:

Two more ways to Bloody Mary bliss:

Bloody Maria: Replace the vodka with tequila, the lemon with lime, and the Tabasco with a teaspoon of canned chipotle pepper.

Asian Mary: Swap the Tabasco for Sriracha and use fish sauce instead of Worcestershire.

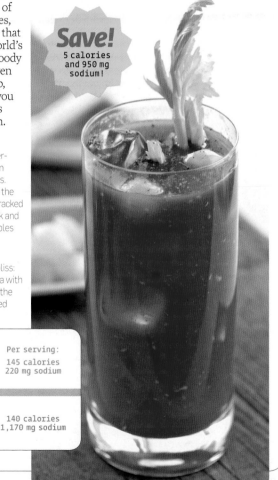

Save!
5 calories and 950 mg sodium!

Per serving:
145 calories
220 mg sodium

140 calories
1,170 mg sodium

Not That!

Red Lobster Bloody Mary

Drink This!
Flavored Latte

Vanilla Latte

2 oz hot espresso
or very strong
coffee

1 Tbsp
sugar-free
vanilla syrup*

½ cup
fat-free milk

* Don't like
vanilla? Try
hazelnut,
chocolate, or
raspberry syrup.
Torani makes a
wide variety of
syrups sweetened
with sucralose,
one of the safest
of the artifi-
cial sweeteners.

www.torani.com

Thanks to Starbucks, lattes have become a common player in the American liquid diet. That doesn't have to be a bad thing, but too often fancy espresso drinks come with huge caloric consequences. By learning to create lattes and cappuccinos at home, you'll save piles of cash and loads of calories over the course of a year. If you don't own a fancy espresso machine, don't fret; the $25 Moka and $15 Bonjour milk frother (see page 224) will have you out-brewing your local barista.

How to Make It:

Combine the espresso and syrup in a coffee mug. Place the milk in a large microwave-safe glass or container. Use a milk frother, moving it up and down slowly in the container for 20 seconds, to create a thick foam (cold milk produces the best foam). Place the milk in the microwave and heat on high for 30 seconds. Add the hot milk to the espresso, then use a spoon to top off the drink with the foam.

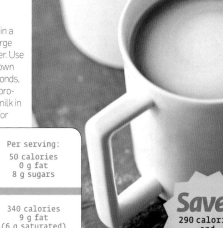

Per serving:
50 calories
0 g fat
8 g sugars

Not That!

Dunkin' Donuts Mocha Raspberry Latte
(medium, 16 fl oz)

340 calories
9 g fat
(6 g saturated)
48 g sugars

Save!
290 calories
and
40 g sugars!

Margarita

In Mexico, the margarita is a simple, perfectly balanced cocktail. Unfortunately, in its travels north of the border, the lime-and-tequila classic picked up a suitcase full of high-fructose corn syrup and with it about 300 extra calories. We've returned it to its simple, unadulterated former self.

The Classic Margarita

1½ oz 100% agave silver tequila

1½ oz fresh lime juice (from about a lime and half), plus extra lime for garnish

1 oz triple sec, Cointreau, or Grand Marnier

1 tsp agave syrup

Coarse salt

How to Make It:

Place the tequila, lime juice, triple sec, and agave syrup in a shaker filled with ice. Cover and shake vigorously for 20 seconds. Cover a small plate with a thin layer of salt. Rub the rim of a rocks glass with the flesh side of a lime wedge, then dip into the salt and crust lightly. Serve in the glass straight up or with ice.

Mix It Up:

Embellishments worth embracing:
Spicy Margarita: Add ½ teaspoon canned chipotle pepper to the shaker. Mix the salt with an equal measure of chili powder for a fiery rim.
Strawberry Margarita: Add four sliced strawberries to the shaker and use a wooden spoon to smash. Proceed with the recipe.

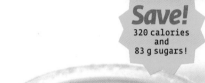

Save!
320 calories
and
83 g sugars!

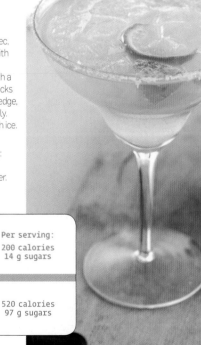

Per serving:
200 calories
14 g sugars

520 calories
97 g sugars

Not That!

**Red Lobster
Top-Shelf Frozen
Margarita**

Drink This!
Sangria

In theory, sangria is a brilliant concept: Up the nutritional ante and stretch a cheap bottle of wine by mixing in fresh fruit. But in the wrong hands, a healthy pour of sangria becomes a glorified glass of fruit punch with double the calories. Thankfully, it's an easy fix, as long as you're playing mixologist.

Red Sangria

1 bottle dry red wine (Don't spend more than $10 on the wine: a light, fruit-forward red like a zinfandel will work perfectly)

½ cup orange juice

1 medium orange, sliced

2 apples (McIntosh works well), peeled and chopped

3 Tbsp superfine sugar

1 cup club soda

Traditional sangria gets a boozy kick from brandy. Feel free to add a splash.

How to Make It:

Combine all of the ingredients except for the club soda in a pitcher and mix to combine. Place in the refrigerator and refrigerate for at least 2 hours or overnight to allow the flavors to marry. When ready to serve, add the club soda. Serve over ice, if you like, with extra orange slices. Makes 8 servings.

Mix It Up:

Two tasty sangria tweaks:

White: Trade the red wine for a bottle of pinot grigio and the apples for a mixture of stone fruit: peaches, plums, and nectarines.

Sparkling: Swap the red for a bottle of Spanish cava or Italian prosecco. Add peaches and cherries.

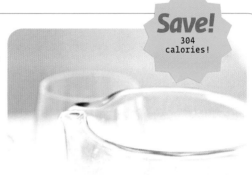

Per serving:
180 calories
16 g sugars

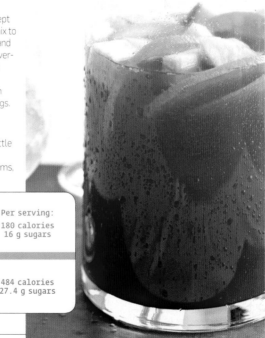

Not That!

Applebee's Red Apple Sangria
(mucho size)

484 calories
27.4 g sugars

Drink This!
Hot Chocolate

Homemade Hot Chocolate

4 cups 2% milk

1 stick cinnamon (plus 4 more for stirring, if you like)

Pinch of nutmeg (preferably freshly ground, which makes all the difference in the world)

2 Tbsp cocoa powder

2 oz dark chocolate, finely chopped

¼ cup sugar

1 tsp vanilla extract

Optional: Pinch of cayenne pepper (trust us, the combo is delicious)

The world of hot chocolate is dominated by two extremes. On one end you have the powder, which may be light in calories but contains a strange brew of additives and scarcely tastes like chocolate. On the other end you have the insanely rich, hyper-caloric stuff served at cafés and restaurants. Our creation fuses the low-calorie potential of that paltry powder with the indulgence of the high-end hot chocolate to create a beautifully balanced treat.

How to Make It:

In a saucepan set over low heat, combine the milk, cinnamon, and nutmeg and simmer for 5 minutes. Remove from heat and stir in the cocoa powder and chopped chocolate. Use a whisk to fully incorporate the chocolate into the milk. When uniformly combined, stir in the sugar and vanilla and whisk again. Return to the heat and cook for another minute until very hot. Serve immediately with a cinnamon stick in each cup for stirring, if you like. Makes 4 servings.

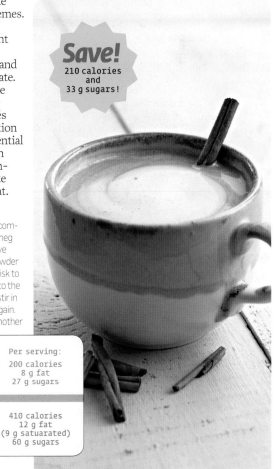

Save!
210 calories and 33 g sugars!

Per serving:
200 calories
8 g fat
27 g sugars

410 calories
12 g fat
(9 g satuarated)
60 g sugars

Not That!

Starbucks White Hot Chocolate
(grande, 16 fl oz)

Blended Coffee Drink

The frozen coffee drink is a costly concoction. A venti Starbucks Frappuccino will run you about $4 in most parts of the country. Drink one four times a week, as many people do, and you're out nearly $1,000 a year. For coffee. But the cost doesn't stop there. At 500 calories a pop, that same Frappuccino addiction will fix an extra 29 pounds on your frame over the course of 365 days. Are you really prepared to pay that steep of a price?

Caramel Coffee Cooler

1 cup strong brewed coffee, cooled

1 cup ice cubes

1 cup 1% milk

¼ cup low-fat vanilla frozen yogurt

1 Tbsp sugar-free caramel syrup

½ Tbsp agave syrup

How to Make It:
Place all the ingredients in a blender and blend until smooth and uniform.

Mix It Up:
Three ways to amp up the flavor:

Chocolate: Replace the caramel with a tablespoon of chocolate sauce (the darker the better) and a pinch of cinnamon.

Banana: Drop a frozen banana into the blender. Continue with the recipe.

Booze: Add a shot of Kahlua or Bailey's to any of the versions above.

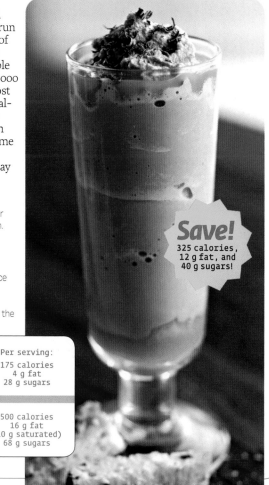

Save!
325 calories, 12 g fat, and 40 g sugars!

Per serving:
175 calories
4 g fat
28 g sugars

500 calories
16 g fat
(10 g saturated)
68 g sugars

Not That!

Starbucks Caramel Frappuccino
(venti, 24 fl oz)

Beer Cocktail

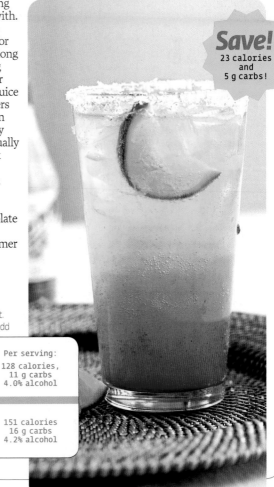

To some, a beer is something that shouldn't be messed with. Fair enough, but mild beers are also the perfect vessel for big flavors. Mexicans have long been in the habit of spiking their beer with a spicy-sour combination of fresh lime juice and hot sauce. Major brewers in the US have picked up on the trend, but unfortunately their take on michelada usually includes stuff you wouldn't want anywhere near your cerveza: high-fructose corn syrup, MSG, and artificial coloring. Make our version once—ideally alongside a plate of grilled fish tacos—and it's guaranteed to be a summer staple for years to come.

Michelada

Coarse salt

Juice of one lime

Ice

1 tsp Worcestershire

1 tsp (or more to taste) hot sauce (Cholula is best)

12 oz bottle Carta Blanca (or any other low-calorie Mexican beer)

Save!
23 calories and 5 g carbs!

How to Make It:

Pour the salt on a plate. Rub the flesh of the squeezed lime around the rim of a glass and dip in the salt. Fill the glass with ice cubes, then add the lime, the Worcestershire, and the hot sauce. Pour in the beer. Drink.

Per serving:
128 calories,
11 g carbs
4.0% alcohol

151 calories
16 g carbs
4.2% alcohol

Not That!

Bud Light & Clamato Chelada

Chai Tea

Over the past decade, chai has gone from an obscure Indian tea known mostly to yogis to the base of one of the most popular coffee-shop drinks in America. As its popularity has grown in café culture, so too has its price and caloric content. Four bucks and 400 calories are standard tolls. That's why we make our own.

Chai Latte

8 whole cloves

1 Tbsp fennel seeds

5 or 6 thin slices fresh ginger

½ Tbsp black peppercorns

1 dried bay leaf

1 cinnamon stick

6 cups water

2 Tbsp black tea, preferably Darjeeling (or 4 bags)

4 Tbsp brown sugar

1½ cups 1% milk

Tweak the blend. Want more heat? Add extra peppercorns. Hate anise? Forget the fennel seeds. It's your world.

How to Make It:

Place the cloves, fennel, ginger, peppercorns, bay leaf, cinnamon stick, and water in a saucepan and bring to a boil. Simmer for 7 minutes, then remove from heat, add the tea, and allow it to steep for 5 minutes. Strain the mixture and return it to the pan. Stir in the brown sugar and milk, bring to a simmer, and once hot all the way through, remove from the heat and serve. Makes 4 servings.

*If you have a milk frother, like the BonJour we recommend on page 224, then you may top this mix with a few spoons of foamy milk and some ground cinnamon.

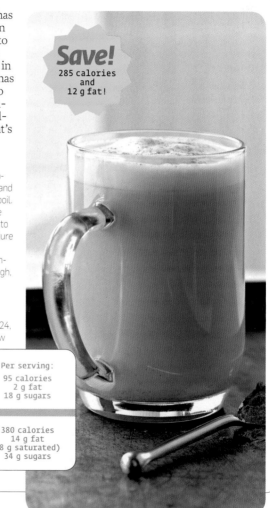

Save!
285 calories and 12 g fat!

Per serving:
95 calories
2 g fat
18 g sugars

Not That!

**Au Bon Pain
Chai Tea Latte**
(medium, 16 oz)

380 calories
14 g fat
(8 g saturated)
34 g sugars

Milk Shake

Peanut Butter Chocolate Shake

1 very ripe banana, frozen

¾ cup fat-free milk

¾ cup low-fat chocolate frozen yogurt (Stonyfield works well)

½ Tbsp peanut butter

3 ice cubes

Milk shakes are the cheese fries of the beverage world. They come bearing catastrophic calorie counts and little to no redeeming nutritional value. Take the Cold Stone PB&C. Do you really want to hop in the car, drive 10 or 15 minutes down the road, wait in a meandering line with a bunch of other sugar junkies, and pony up your hard-earned cash for a drink that will wipe out your entire day's caloric allotment? Or you could break out the blender and spend 90 seconds of your day making a decadent shake that will save you three or four bucks and the caloric equivalent of three Big Macs. Which would you prefer? Yeah, us too.

How to Make It:
Combine all of the ingredients in a blender and blend until smooth and uniform.

Save!
1,660 calories
and
103 g sugars!

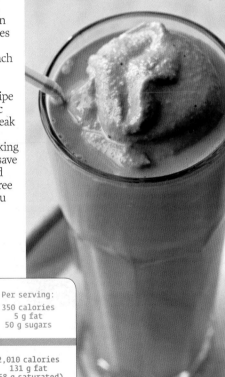

Per serving:
350 calories
5 g fat
50 g sugars

 Not That!

Cold Stone Creamery PB&C Shake
(Gotta Have It size, 24 fl oz)

2,010 calories
131 g fat
(68 g saturated)
153 g sugars

A&W

D+ Drink Report Card

C- Food Report Card

● A&W isn't just docked because their namesake brew is one of the sweetest beverages on the planet. No, the real issue here is a menu utterly devoid of any real nutrition. Where's the juice? The milk? The tea? Nowhere to be found. Sadly, the food menu suffers a similar fate, littered as it is with burgers, trans fat-laden sides, and little else.

For 880 calories, you can have

ALL THIS

A Coney Dog, Regular Corn Dog Nuggets, and a Vanilla Ice Cream Cone

OR

THAT

A Medium Chocolate Milk Shake

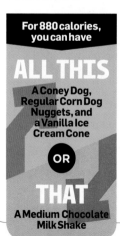

Drink This

A&W Root Beer Float

(small, 16 fl oz)

330 calories
5 g fat
(3 g saturated)
57 g sugars

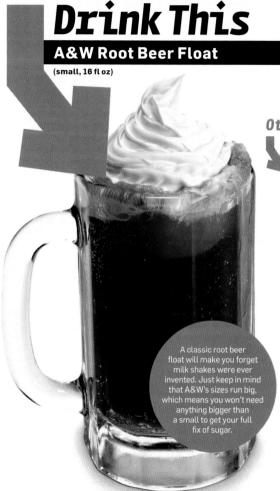

A classic root beer float will make you forget milk shakes were ever invented. Just keep in mind that A&W's sizes run big, which means you won't need anything bigger than a small to get your full fix of sugar.

Other Picks

A&W Diet Root Beer Float
(20 fl oz)
170 calories
5 g fat
(3 g saturated)
17 g sugars

Lipton Raspberry Iced Tea
(medium, 14 fl oz)
140 calories
0 g fat
37 g sugars

Vanilla Cone
250 calories
7 g fat
(5 g saturated)
27 g sugars

50

430 calories
9 g fat
(5 g saturated)
37 g sugars

Not That!
A&W Root Beer Freeze
(small, 16 fl oz)

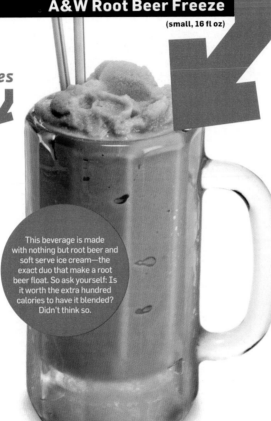

This beverage is made with nothing but root beer and soft serve ice cream—the exact duo that make a root beer float. So ask yourself: Is it worth the extra hundred calories to have it blended? Didn't think so.

Other Passes

A&W Regular Root Beer
(14 fl oz)
290 calories
0 g fat
76 g sugars

Wild Cherry Pepsi
(medium, 14 fl oz)
180 calories
0 g fat
49 g sugars

Oreo Polar Swirl
(small, 12 fl oz)
720 calories
32 g fat
(15 g saturated)
104 g sugars

WEAPON OF MASS DESTRUCTION
Large Vanilla Milk Shake
(32 fl oz)

1,150 calories
50 g fat
(30 g saturated)
91 g sugars

This full-fat ice cream is spiked with corn-based sweeteners and topped with a mountain of whipped cream. The result weighs in heavier than 10 scoops of Breyers All Natural French Vanilla Ice Cream. If you want a cold treat, make it a small float or a cone.

GUILTY PLEASURE

Chocolate Sundae

320 calories
8 g fat
15 g sugars

It might not be a drink, but it's definitely cold, sweet, and refreshing. Plus, with the exception of the Diet Root Beer Float, it has fewer calories than any frozen drink on the menu.

APPLEBEE'S

C-	D+
Drink Report Card	Food Report Card

● Even if you manage to look past the sangrias, martinis, and margaritas that occupy most of the real estate on Applebee's beverage menu, there's still a whole list of smoothies, shakes, and citrus-flavored sodas to draw you in. Nonetheless, a C- is a small improvement over its food grade, which houses over two dozen dishes with more than 1,000 calories, including the dreaded Riblets.

HIDDEN DANGER

Oriental Chicken Salad

It's hard to pick just one hidden danger here, but a bowl of "fresh Asian greens" that eats up 71 percent of your day's calories is especially perilous.

**1,430 calories
1,920 mg sodium**

Drink This
Mochatini

160 calories

Applebee's refuses to offer full nutritional information for its menu items

Consider this the most decadent cocktail you'll ever find with fewer than 200 calories. It's made with a combination of Starbucks' Coffee and Godiva Chocolate liqueurs blended with vanilla vodka and a splash of cream.

Other Picks

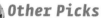

Jack & Coke
110 calories

Mango Martini
190 calories

Mango Banana Smoothie
260-360 calories

540 calories

Not That!
Applebee's Mud Slide

Other Passes

Red Apple Sangria
240 calories

Mango Main Street Rita Swirl
500 calories

Mango Shake
820-1,000 calories

Applebee's mudslide rendition would be better thought of as an over-size ice cream sundae with a splash of Kahlua on top. Somehow the combo yields a cocktail with 210 calories more than McDonald's Hot Fudge Sundae.

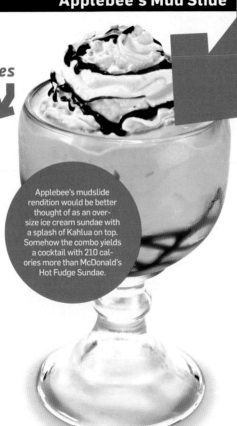

PERFECT PARTNER

9 oz House Sirloin with Seasonal Vegetables
390 calories

A steak this lean is hard to come by, especially at a place like Applebee's, where everything tends to pack more calories. Plus, if your drink of choice is alcoholic, the steak's protein will slow the alcohol's absorption, keeping your blood sugar stable and you standing upright.

For 500 calories, you can have

ALL THIS

A Cajun Lime Tilapia Entrée with Black Bean and Corn Salsa, Rice Pilaf, Seasoned Vegetables, and a Mango Martini

OR

THAT

A Main Street Wildberry 'Rita

AU BON PAIN

C+	A-
Drink Report Card	Food Report Card

● Au Bon Pain serves up a diverse range of coffee drinks, juices, and smoothies. But those options are sometimes difficult to find amid Au Bon's long list of cloying teas, syrupy mochas, and ice cream blasts. Avoid the extra calories by ordering drinks you know— juice, cappuccinos, and regular lattes.

Drink This

Iced Chai Latte
(medium, 16 fl oz)

260 calories
7 g fat
(5 g saturated)
25 g sugars

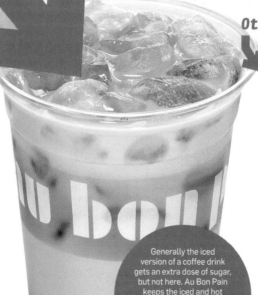

Generally the iced version of a coffee drink gets an extra dose of sugar, but not here. Au Bon Pain keeps the iced and hot ingredients the same, which allows the ice in the cup to offset a load of superfluous calories from sugar and fat.

Other Picks

Vanilla Americano
(large, 20 fl oz)
75 calories
0 g fat
17 g sugars

Strawberry Smoothie
(medium, 16 fl oz)
310 calories
1 g fat
(0 g saturated)
43 g sugars

Iced French Vanilla Coffee
(large, 28 fl oz)
15 calories
0 g fat
(0 g saturated)
0 g sugars

For 760 calories, you can have

ALL THIS
A Chocolate-Dipped Cranberry Almond Macaroon, Mango Coconut Mousse, and a Small Iced Caramel Macchiato

OR

THAT
A Large Vanilla Blast
(24 fl oz)

380 calories
14 g fat
(8 g saturated)
34 g sugars

Not That!

Chai Latte
(medium, 16 fl oz)

Other Passes

Vanilla Latte
(large, 20 fl oz)
500 calories
14 g fat
(9 g saturated)
81 g sugars

Vanilla Blast
(medium, 16 fl oz)
540 calories
17 g fat
(15 g saturated)
99 g sugars

Iced Vanilla Latte
(small, 12 fl oz)
240 calories
5 g fat
(3 g saturated)
44 g sugars

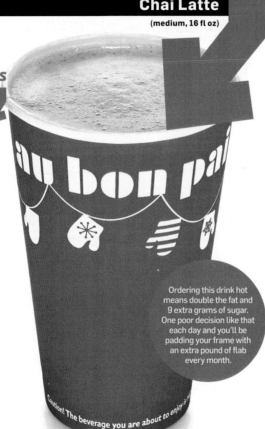

Caution! The beverage you are about to enjoy is

Ordering this drink hot means double the fat and 9 extra grams of sugar. One poor decision like that each day and you'll be padding your frame with an extra pound of flab every month.

PERFECT PARTNER

Perfect Portion Menu
70-200 calories

This snack-driven selection from Au Bon Pain is one of our favorite menu concepts in America. All 16 options offer big flavor in a compact package for 200 calories or less. One makes a great companion to an afternoon cup of coffee or tea, or combine two for a near-perfect lunch. Our favorite combo? The Chicken Pesto Salad and Watermelon, Almonds, and Feta.

HIDDEN DANGER

Medium Hot Chocolate
(16 fl oz)

Hot chocolates are always dangerous on-the-go drinks, but this one, made with whole milk and a barrage of sweeteners, is the worst of all.

460 calories
15 g fat
(9 g saturated)
68 g sugar

AUNTIE ANNE'S

● Auntie Anne's serves up 29 different shakes, slushes, smoothies, and sweetened lattes. She balances that with a handful of teas by Nestea and Gold Peak. But when it comes to pretzel pairings, there's nothing more perfect than a regular cup of joe. Fortunately they have that, too.

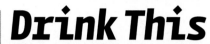

Drink This
Blue Raspberry Icee

(21 fl oz)

160 calories
0 g fat
41 g sugars

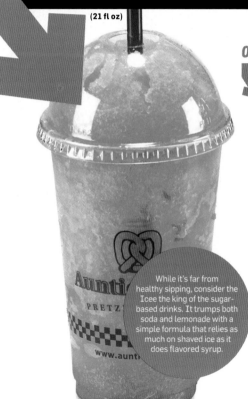

While it's far from healthy sipping, consider the Icee the king of the sugar-based drinks. It trumps both soda and lemonade with a simple formula that relies as much on shaved ice as it does flavored syrup.

SUGAR SP✦KE

Large Hi-C Fruit Punch
(42 oz)

The Impact:
104 GRAMS!

Despite the similarity of the names, "fruit punch" and "fruit juice" are entirely different animals. Punch may disguise itself as something vaguely fruit-based, but rarely does it contain anything even resembling real fruit.

Other Picks

Strawberry Dutch Ice
(14 fl oz)
160 calories
0 g fat
(0 g saturated)
37 g sugars

Coffee Dutch Latte
(14 fl oz)
290 calories
14 g fat
(9 g saturated)
34 g sugars

Kiwi-Banana Dutch Smoothie
(14 fl oz)
270 calories
10 g fat
(7 g saturated)
38 g sugars

310 calories
0 g fat
73 g sugars

Not That!

Lemonade Mixer Blue Raspberry

(20 fl oz)

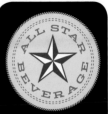

Gold Peak Sweetened Green Tea (16 fl oz)

130 calories
34 g sugars

Unlike 90% of restaurant beverages, tea—even the sweetened stuff—offers nutritional rewards in the form of free-radical eradicating flavonoids and polyphenols. Together these can help boost your metabolism and defend your body from certain cancers.

Other Passes

Strawberry Dutch Shake

(14 fl oz)

600 calories
27 g fat
(18 g saturated)
73 g sugars

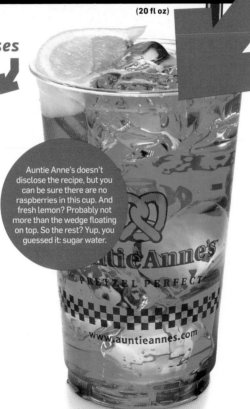

Auntie Anne's doesn't disclose the recipe, but you can be sure there are no raspberries in this cup. And fresh lemon? Probably not more than the wedge floating on top. So the rest? Yup, you guessed it: sugar water.

Mocha Dutch Latte

(14 fl oz)

360 calories
17 g fat
(11 g saturated)
38 g sugars

Piña Colada Dutch Smoothie

(20 fl oz)

470 calories
15 g fat
(10 g saturated)
75 g sugars

SIZE MATTERS!

STRAWBERRY LEMONADE

LARGE

(42 fl oz)
570 calories

small

(16 fl oz)
210 calories

Total Savings: 360 CALORIES!

57

BOB EVANS

A	C
Drink Report Card	Food Report Card

● Bob's beverage menu boasts all the options that you should be working into your diet on a regular basis: green and black teas, milk, and a variety of juices. Couple that with a handful of lightly sweetened flavored teas and you have the makings of one of America's best beverage programs.

HIDDEN DANGER

Large Tomato Juice
(14.4 fl oz)

Tomato juice can be an excellent low-calorie alternative to OJ, but not when a single glass contains more sodium than you'd find in 8 small bags of Lay's potato chips.

69 calories
1,474 mg sodium

Drink This
Arnold Palmer
(20 fl oz)

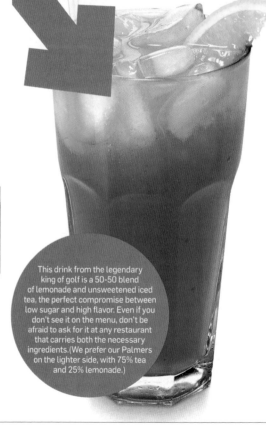

This drink from the legendary king of golf is a 50-50 blend of lemonade and unsweetened iced tea, the perfect compromise between low sugar and high flavor. Even if you don't see it on the menu, don't be afraid to ask for it at any restaurant that carries both the necessary ingredients.(We prefer our Palmers on the lighter side, with 75% tea and 25% lemonade.)

85 calories
0 g fat
20 g sugars

Other Picks

Chocolate Milk
(large, 14.5 fl oz)
280 calories
4 g fat
(0 g saturated)
49 g sugars

Wild Raspberry Iced Tea
(17.6 fl oz)
81 calories
0 g fat
14 g sugars

Caramel Iced Coffee
(10.6 fl oz)
104 calories
4 g fat
(3 g saturated)
15 g sugars

134 calories
0 g fat
32 g sugars

Not That!
Lemonade
(large, 12 fl oz)

Other Passes

Candy Cane Hot Chocolate
(13.5 fl oz)
478 calories
14 g fat
(13 g saturated)
121 g sugars

Wild Raspberry Lemonade
(17.6 fl oz)
215 calories
0 g fat
19 g sugars

Caramel Mocha
(10.9 fl oz)
268 calories
9 g fat
(8 g saturated)
41 g sugars

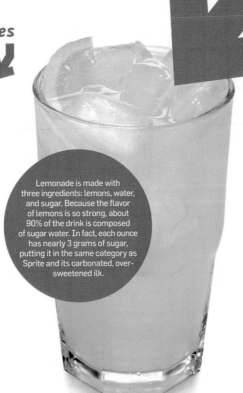

Lemonade is made with three ingredients: lemons, water, and sugar. Because the flavor of lemons is so strong, about 90% of the drink is composed of sugar water. In fact, each ounce has nearly 3 grams of sugar, putting it in the same category as Sprite and its carbonated, over-sweetened ilk.

PERFECT PARTNER

Wildfire Salmon
244 calories
9 g fat
(2 g saturated)
203 mg sodium

Not only is this the best option on all of Bob's menu, it qualifies as one of the healthiest entrées in all of America. Nearly every calorie of this spicy salmon dish comes from healthy omega-3 fats or from the astounding 41 grams of protein.

BEVERAGE MYTH

Juice is healthier than milk.

Milk and juice are calorically similar, but while juice earns its calories entirely from sugar, milk's calories come from a distribution of sugar, fat, and protein, which means it takes longer to digest and provides your body with all the essential amino acids. Furthermore, milk is loaded with iodine, vitamin D, and vitamin B_2. That's not to say fruit juice is bad, just that cow juice is better.

BURGER KING

● Sure, the King sells coffee, juice, and milk, but the bulk of BK's menu consists of sodas, Icees, and milk shakes. The result is a beverage lineup that mirrors its food offerings: a few bright spots amid a cast of underachievers.

GUILTY PLEASURE

Whopper Jr

340 calories
20 g fat (5 g saturated)
530 mg sodium

We've long been fans of the Whopper, just not the bigger versions, which carry anywhere from 670 calories to more than 1,200 for a Triple with Cheese. The Whopper Jr., however, delivers a nice dose of protein, plus a decent bit of vegetation, for 100 calories fewer than the medium french fries. Nix the mayo and save an extra 80 calories and 9 grams of fat.

Drink This

Chocolate Milk Shake

(value size, 12 fl oz)

310 calories
9 g fat
(7 g saturated)
51 g sugars

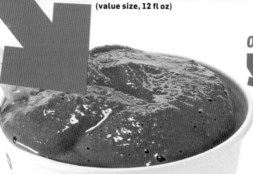

When you start to recognize a shake as a dessert, not a thirst-quencher, you'll start to realize that you never need more than 12 ounces—and often you can get by with even less. This chocolate version from the King is one of the lowest calorie shakes we've seen.

Other Picks

Icee Coca-Cola/ Frozen Coke
(22 fl oz)
140 calories
0 g fat
40 g sugars

Hershey's 1% Chocolate Milk
(8 fl oz)
180 calories
2.5 g fat
(1.5 g saturated)
29 g sugars

Icee Cherry
(22 fl oz)
140 calories
0 g fat
40 g sugars

700 calories
26 g fat
(16 g saturated,
0.5 g trans)
105 g sugars

Not That!

Chocolate Oreo BK Sundae Shake

(value size, 16 fl oz)

Other Passes

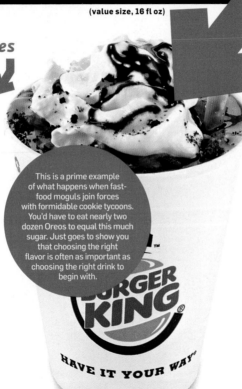

Coca-Cola Classic
(medium, 22 fl oz)
210 calories
0 g fat
56 g sugars

Mocha BK Joe Iced Coffee
(22 fl oz)
360 calories
10 g fat
(6 g saturated)
63 g sugars

Strawberry Milk Shake
(medium, 22 fl oz)
630 calories
15 g fat
(11 g saturated)
102 g sugars

This is a prime example of what happens when fast-food moguls join forces with formidable cookie tycoons. You'd have to eat nearly two dozen Oreos to equal this much sugar. Just goes to show you that choosing the right flavor is often as important as choosing the right drink to begin with.

124
The number of times you would have to push a lawnmower from one end zone to the other on a football field in order to burn off the 1,010 calories in a large Oreo BK Chocolate Sundae Shake

CHEESECAKE FACTORY

Drink This

Peach Smoothie

199 calories
0 g saturated fat
48 g carbs

● We're thankful that the beverage side of the menu is healthier than the Cheesecake Factory's food selections. But sadly, that's not saying much. The beverage lineup is long on cocktails and sugary coffee concoctions and short on safe, simple low-calorie drinks. Smoothies, unsweetened tea, and, of course, water, are your best bets.

66

The number of alcoholic beverages on Cheesecake Factory's menu for which they have yet to provide any nutritional information

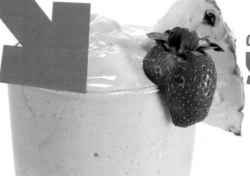

Cheesecake Factory refuses to offer full nutritional information for its menu items

Not even the small peach smoothies at Jamba Juice weigh in with such a modest load of calories. An unexpected high point of what may be America's Unhealthiest Restaurant.

Other Picks

White Chocolate Raspberry Latte
339 calories
7 g saturated fat
55 g carbs

Cold Apple Cider
165 calories
0 g fat
42 g carbs

Cappuccino
79 calories
3 g saturated fat
7 g carbs

346 calories
3 g saturated fat
76 g carbs

Not That!
Frozen Iced Mango

Other Passes

Factory Hot Chocolate
547 calories
19 g saturated fat
58 g carbs

Strawberry Lemonade
196 calories
0 g fat
48 g carbs

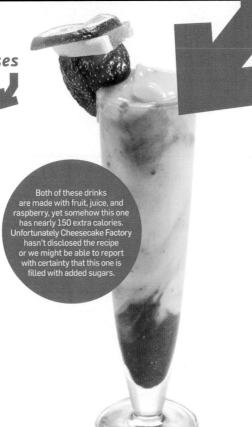

Both of these drinks are made with fruit, juice, and raspberry, yet somehow this one has nearly 150 extra calories. Unfortunately Cheesecake Factory hasn't disclosed the recipe or we might be able to report with certainty that this one is filled with added sugars.

Café Mocha
424 calories
17 g saturated fat
35 g carbs

WEAPON OF MASS DESTRUCTION
Bistro Shrimp Pasta

2,819 calories
77 g saturated fat
184 g carbohydrates

This is a book about beverages, but we'd be remiss not to point out this pasta, currently the Worst Food in America. The innocuous-sounding name obscures the fact that tussling with this plate of glorified shrimp Alfredo is like sitting down to a dinner of 14 Krispy Kreme Doughnuts.

PERFECT PARTNER

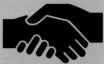

Edamame
323 calories
0 g saturated fat

Need something to chew on while you're sharing a drink with friends? These salted soybeans are loaded with protein, and the simple act of working them from their pods will keep your mind off the Factory's long menu of 1,000-calorie appetizers.

CHEVY'S FRESH MEX

D+ Drink Report Card

D Food Report Card

Drink This
Mango Mojito

190 calories

● Chevy's effort to entice you with high-dollar cocktails comes at the cost of more nutritious beverage options, which is especially problematic considering it's also difficult to find an entrée with fewer than 1,000 calories. So here's your strategy: If you want alcohol, make it a light beer or a mojito. If you're not tippling, then it's tea or water, okay?

KILLER APP

Guacamole
(7 oz)
300 calories
26 g fat
(4 g saturated)
380 mg sodium

If you're looking for a healthy, hunger-fighting appetizer, there's nothing better than guac. Avocadoes are loaded with fiber and cholesterol-lowering monounsaturated fats, both of which digest slowly so that they stay in your stomach longer.

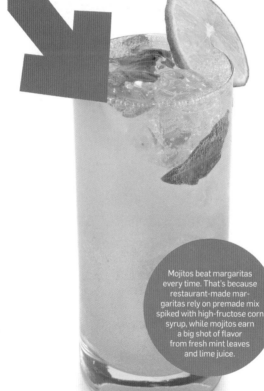

Mojitos beat margaritas every time. That's because restaurant-made margaritas rely on premade mix spiked with high-fructose corn syrup, while mojitos earn a big shot of flavor from fresh mint leaves and lime juice.

Other Picks

Lipton Iced Tea with Lemon Wedge
(10 fl oz)
0 calories
0 g fat
0 g sugars

Cosmopolitan
180 calories

Modelo Especial
(1 bottle, 12 fl oz)
145 calories

64

460 calories

Not That!
Spicy Mango Margarita

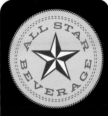

Red Wine
100-150 calories

At a restaurant awash in sugary margaritas, consider red wine your life perserver. The antioxidants in the grape skins have been shown to fight off long-term degenerative diseases such as cancer and heart disease.

Other Passes

Brisk Raspberry Iced Tea
(10 fl oz)
110 calories
0 g fat
29 g sugars

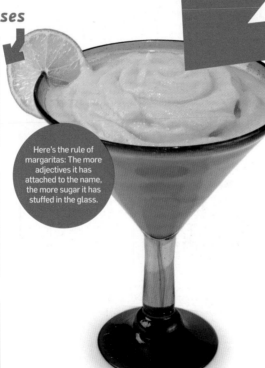

Here's the rule of margaritas: The more adjectives it has attached to the name, the more sugar it has stuffed in the glass.

Pomegranate Martini
320 calories

Negro Modelo
(1 bottle, 12 fl oz)
169 calories

BEVERAGE MYTH

Liquor before beer, you're in the clear.

Followed this one before? Still felt lousy the next day? Well you shouldn't be surprised; the old "beer before liquor" maxim is one with no science to support it. The rationale is that it's easier to moderate your drinking when you finish the night with lower-alcohol beer rather than switching to higher-alcohol hooch, but the truth is, it's how much and how fast you drink that determines your buzz, not the order in which you do it.

CHILI'S

● Sure, Chili's beverage menu skews slightly toward the alcoholic options, yet despite the disadvantage, they still manage to minimize the number of calorie bombs. About half of the signature cocktails on the menu fall below 300 calories, but what's better are the nonalcoholic drinks, which include lightly sweetened blackberry and mango iced teas alongside the usual coffee, milk, and juice options.

Drink This
Presidente Margarita

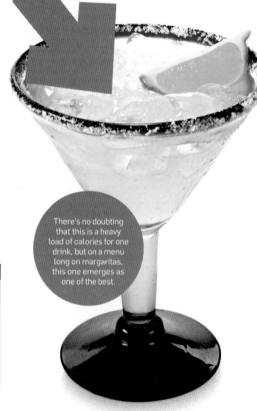

There's no doubting that this is a heavy load of calories for one drink, but on a menu long on margaritas, this one emerges as one of the best.

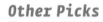

240 calories

Other Picks

Mango Iced Tea
15 calories

Top Shelf Margarita
260 calories

Grand Patron Margarita
230 calories

FOOD COURT

THE CRIME
Bottomless Coke with two refills
(450 calories)

THE PUNISHMENT
Climb 1,665 steps, the height of the Eiffel Tower

410 calories

Not That!
El Niño Margarita

Other Passes

Strawberry Lemonade
100 calories

Frozen Top Shelf Margaritas
(strawberry mango, strawberry, raspberry, or mango)
330-410 calories

Blue Pacific Margarita
330 calories

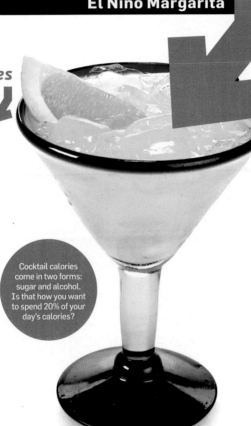

Cocktail calories come in two forms: sugar and alcohol. Is that how you want to spend 20% of your day's calories?

MARGARITA DECODER
(Listed best to worst)

PRESIDENTE MARGARITA: Tequila and Cointreau flavored with Presidente Brandy, a Mexican grape brandy with a delicate fruity flavor

TROPICAL SUNRISE MARGARITA: Tequila and melon liqueur flavored with pineapple juice and a splash of grenadine

BLUE PACIFIC MARGARITA: Tequila and Cointreau flavored with Blue Curacao, a candy sweet liqueur made from the dried peels of bitter oranges

EL NIÑO MARGARITA: Tequila and Cointreau flavored with fresh orange juice and GranGala, an orange liqueur that packs on excess sugar and calories

COSI

C Drink Report Card

B Food Report Card

● Cosi's menu has two faces. One is harmless, offering low-calorie drinks like Americanos, iced teas, and cups of soymilk. The other face is more vicious; it turns average drinks into liabilities (15-ounce mochas with more than 400 calories?) and monstrous drinks into belt-line expanders (like the 1,200-calorie Double Oh! Arctic Mocha).

For 1,210 calories, you can have

ALL THIS

A Tuscan Pesto Chicken Sandwich, Chocolate and Marshmallow S'mores, and a Tall Arctic Mocha

OR

THAT

Gigante Double Oh! Arctic Mocha (23 fl oz)

Drink This

Raspberry Iced Tea

(gigante, 20 fl oz)

125 calories
0 g fat
30 g carbs

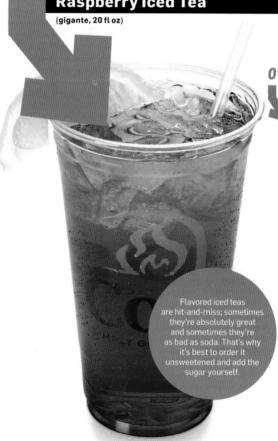

Flavored iced teas are hit-and-miss; sometimes they're absolutely great and sometimes they're as bad as soda. That's why it's best to order it unsweetened and add the sugar yourself.

Other Picks

Cafe Au Lait
(grande, 15 fl oz)
145 calories
5 g fat
(5 g saturated)
12 g carbs

Chocolate Covered Strawberry Smoothie
(grande, 15 fl oz)
419 calories
17 g fat
(10 g saturated)
62 g carbs

Chai Tea Latte
(grande, 15 fl oz)
214 calories
8 g fat
(5 g saturated)
29 g carbs

399 calories
0 g fat
80 g carbs

Not That!

Raspberry Mojito Lemonade

(gigante, 20 fl oz)

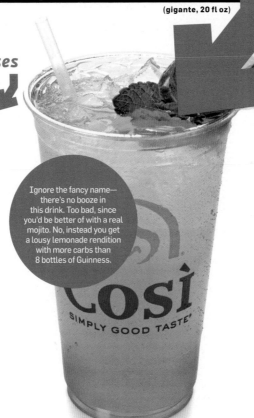

SIMPLY GOOD TASTE

Ignore the fancy name—there's no booze in this drink. Too bad, since you'd be better of with a real mojito. No, instead you get a lousy lemonade rendition with more carbs than 8 bottles of Guinness.

Other Passes

Mocha
(grande, 15 fl oz)
411 calories
10 g fat
(6 g saturated)
68 g carbs

Double Oh! Arctic
(grande, 15 fl oz)
892 calories
19 g fat
(10 g saturated)
180 g carbs

Citrus Passion Fruit Smoothie
(grande, 15 fl oz)
420 calories
0 g fat
85 g carbs

BEVERAGE MYTH

Soda is the most concentrated source of sugar in our diets.

There's no denying the fact that soda is an evil force in the American diet, but there are worse sugar offenders at work. Consider this: A 12-ounce soda has about 40 grams of sugar. The same size serving of both Cosi's Raspberry Mojito Lemonade and Mocha have about 45 grams of sugar each, nearly all of it added. That's no excuse to have a soft drink; it's just a warning that sugar comes in many different disguises.

DENNY'S

B-	C
Drink Report Card	Food Report Card

● Denny's gets downgraded for a handful of indulgent selections such as the Cherry Cherry Limeade, Strawberry Mango Pucker, and infamous Oreo Blender Blaster. But the menu is balanced with a choice list of lightly sweetened iced teas, milk, and less-common but healthier juices such as grape-fruit and tomato.

HIDDEN DANGER

Double Cheeseburger

No one should be surprised to see that a bi-pattied package is bad for them. But this one is laced with nearly four days' worth of trans fat, making it America's Most Dangerous Burger.

1,540 calories
116 g fat
(52 g saturated,
7 g trans)
3,880 mg sodium

Drink This

Root Beer Float

(16 fl oz)

430 calories
17 g fat
(9 g saturated)
63 g sugars

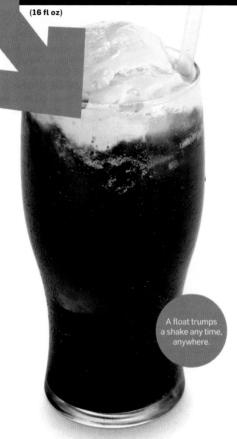

A float trumps a shake any time, anywhere.

Other Picks

Blueberry Pomegranate Tea Chiller
(15 fl oz)
120 calories
0 g fat
29 g sugars

Orange Juice
(10 fl oz)
140 calories
0 g fat
30 g sugars

Lemonade
(16 fl oz)
150 calories
0 g fat
31 g sugars

890 calories
44 g fat
(20 g saturated)
77 g sugars

Not That!

Oreo Blender Blaster

(14 fl oz)

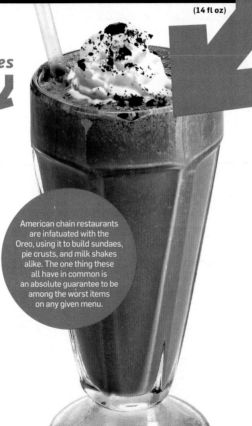

Other Passes

Cranberry Juice
(10 fl oz)
160 calories
0 g fat
40 g sugars

OJ Strawberry Mango
(14 fl oz)
250 calories
0 g fat
56 g sugars

Strawberry Mango Pucker
(15 fl oz)
220 calories
0 g fat
52 g sugars

American chain restaurants are infatuated with the Oreo, using it to build sundaes, pie crusts, and milk shakes alike. The one thing these all have in common is an absolute guarantee to be among the worst items on any given menu.

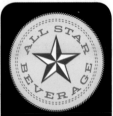

Ruby Red Grapefruit Juice
(10 fl oz)
164 calories
36 g sugars

Americans drink five times more apple juice than grapefruit juice, yet grapefruits are the more nutritious of the two. They have more of nearly every micronutrient, including about 40 times more vitamin C. Make the switch.

GUILTY PLEASURE

Hot Chocolate
(8 fl oz)
100 calories
2 g fat (2 g saturated)
24 g sugars

If calories were currency, you probably wouldn't want to pay for most of the desserts on Denny's menu: 830 calories for a hot fudge brownie; 820 for carrot cake. Hot chocolate, on the other hand, is a treat you can actually afford.

EINSTEIN BROS./NOAH'S BAGELS

● Both Einstein Bros. and Noah's are owned by the Einstein Noah Restaurant Group, and like other coffee purveyors, they give you much control over how your drink is put together. Use only skim milk and sugar-free syrup and you drastically cut calories; if you stick to the standard formulas, you might find yourself sipping a meal's worth of calories.

GUILTY PLEASURE

Iced Mocha
(16 fl oz)

210 calories
6 g fat (4 g saturated)
31 g sugars

Two incentives for asking to have your mocha poured over ice: 1) The ice cubes take the place of what would otherwise be more sugar in your cup; and 2) It turns your drink into the perfect hot-weather treat. Enjoy.

Drink This

Wild Berry Frozen Blended Drink
(18 fl oz)

290 calories
0 g fat
50 g sugars

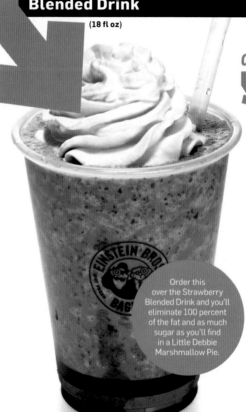

Order this over the Strawberry Blended Drink and you'll eliminate 100 percent of the fat and as much sugar as you'll find in a Little Debbie Marshmallow Pie.

Other Picks

Spontaneitea
(24 fl oz)
100 calories
0 g fat
25 g sugars

Cappuccino
(regular, 12 fl oz)
90 calories
3.5 g fat
(2 g saturated)
8 g sugars

Fat-Free Café Latte
with a pump of caramel syrup (large, 20 fl oz)
280 calories
1 g fat
(0.5 g saturated)
48 g sugars

450 calories
19 g fat
(14 g saturated)
64 g sugars

Not That!

Strawberry Blended Drink
(18 fl oz)

Other Passes

Lemonade Blackberry
(16 fl oz)
310 calories
0 g fat
74 g sugars

Café Latte
(regular, 12 fl oz)
140 calories
5 g fat
(3.5 g saturated)
13 g sugars

Mocha
(15 fl oz)
390 calories
20 g fat
(12 g saturated)
38 g sugars

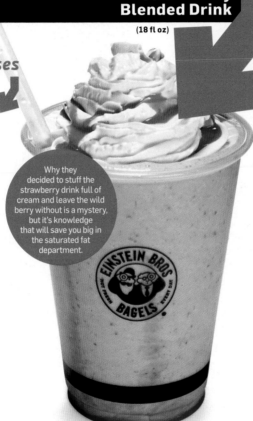

Why they decided to stuff the strawberry drink full of cream and leave the wild berry without is a mystery, but it's knowledge that will save you big in the saturated fat department.

EINSTEIN BROS BAGELS

SUGAR SP KE

Large Chai Tea with Fat-Free Milk
(20 fl oz)

The Impact:
75 GRAMS!

In some eastern countries, "chai" is synonymous with "tea." In America, however, chai denotes black tea that is spiced and flavored however each particular coffeehouse decides. Einstein begins its with a "chai tea concentrate" that packs more sugar than four of their Cinnamon Walnut Strudels.

For 870 calories, you can have

ALL THIS

Hazelnut Iced Coffee, Baked Apple Pie, Hot Fudge Sundae, Oatmeal Raisin Cookie, and Fruit 'n Yogurt Parfait

OR

THAT

A Large (24 fl oz) Cookies and Cream Frozen Blended Drink

B+
Drink
Report
Card

C+
Food
Report
Card

● Jack in the Box has three main flaws. First, it offers a "value-meal" beverage incentive, which rewards you for drinking soda. Second, the large soda is a full 44 ounces—as big as it gets in the restaurant industry. And finally, the large milk shakes can have more than 1,400 calories. But fortunately these problems are avoidable, as Jack also offers milk, juice, iced coffee, tea, and real fruit smoothies. On the solid side of things, after we harped on them for years, Jack has finally removed trans fat from its frying oil—one of the last chains to do so. Thank you! But beware: The burgers are still heavy on the nasty stuff.

Eat This

Chocolate Overload Cake

(1 slice)

300 calories
7 g fat
(1.5 g saturated)
34 g sugars

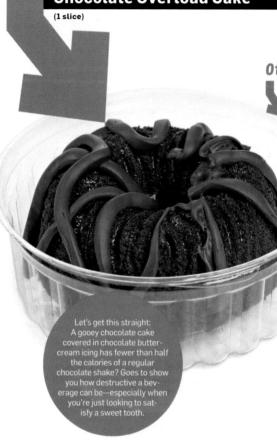

Let's get this straight: A gooey chocolate cake covered in chocolate buttercream icing has fewer than half the calories of a regular chocolate shake? Goes to show you how destructive a beverage can be—especially when you're just looking to satisfy a sweet tooth.

Other Picks

2% Milk Chug
(8 fl oz)
130 calories
5 g fat
(3 g saturated)
13 g sugars
10 g protein

Pomegranate-Berry Smoothie
(16 fl oz)
280 calories
0g fat
(0 g saturated)
53 g sugars

Iced Caramel Coffee
(16 fl oz)
94 calories
1.5 g fat
(1 g saturated)
16 g sugars

750 calories
36 g fat
(24 g saturated,
1.5 g trans)
84 g sugars

Not That!
Chocolate Ice Cream Shake
(16 fl oz)

Other Passes

Orange Juice
(10 fl oz)
140 calories
0 g fat
27 g sugars
0 g protein

Strawberry Ice Cream Shake
(24 fl oz)
730 calories
35 g fat
(24 g saturated,
2 g trans)
76 g sugars

Coca-Cola Classic
(20 fl oz)
170 calories
0 g fat
46 g sugars

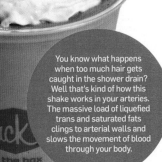

You know what happens when too much hair gets caught in the shower drain? Well that's kind of how this shake works in your arteries. The massive load of liquefied trans and saturated fats clings to arterial walls and slows the movement of blood through your body.

PERFECT PARTNER

Chicken Fajita Pita with Fire-Roasted Salsa
331 calories
10 g fat (6 g saturated)
1,092 mg sodium

Jack's pita is easily the healthiest item on its food menu. Aside from cheese and chicken, the whole-grain shell is filled with lettuce, tomato, and grilled onions. The best part? Chunky salsa.

HIDDEN DANGER

Large Minute Maid Lemonade **(44 fl oz)**
Lemons are harmless citrus fruits; Minute Maid is a respected brand. How bad could this be, right? This cup contains only 3% juice, and the remaining calories are a combination of sugar and HFCS, making lemonade a closer relative to soda than juice.

345 calories
89 g sugars

75

McDONALD'S

● Mickey D's deserves credit for being one of the country's most-improved restaurants. Not only has it introduced healthier food options, but it's also rolled out the McCafe, Ronald's hat in the proverbial coffee ring. Even though it sells lots of zero-calorie coffee and juice, it also pushes plenty of high-sugar caffeine kicks, bottomless sodas, and one of the country's worst milkshake lines.

Drink This

Iced Latte

with nonfat milk and two sugar packets (medium, 16 fl oz)

90 calories
0 g fat
17 g sugars

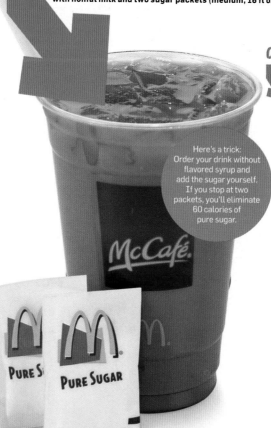

Here's a trick: Order your drink without flavored syrup and add the sugar yourself. If you stop at two packets, you'll eliminate 60 calories of pure sugar.

Other Picks

Orange Juice
(medium, 16 fl oz)
180 calories
0 g fat
37 g sugars

Fat-Free Caramel Cappuccino
(medium, 16 fl oz)
190 calories
0 g fat
41 g sugars

Hot Fudge Sundae
330 calories
10 g fat
(7 g saturated)
48 g sugars

1,905

The number of sit-ups you would have to do to burn off the 1,160 calories in a 32-ounce Chocolate Triple Thick Shake

200 calories
8 g fat
(5 g saturated)
30 g sugars

Not That!

Iced Coffee
(medium, 11.5 fl oz)

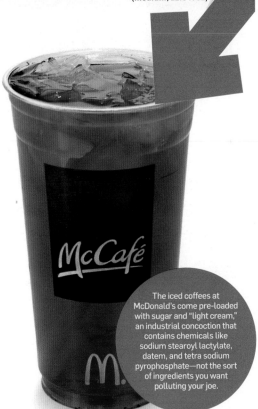

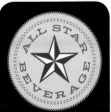

Small Coffee
(12 fl oz)

0 calories
0 g fat
0 g sugars

Forget the antiquated idea that coffee is bad for you. Recent studies have shown that habitual coffee drinkers are half as likely to die of heart disease, develop Parkinson's disease, or develop diabetes. And here's a reason to drink up at McDonald's: In a *Consumer Reports* taste test, it outranked Starbucks, Dunkin' Donuts, and Burger King.

Other Passes

Hi-C Orange Lavaburst
(medium, 21 fl oz)
240 calories
0 g fat
64 g sugars

Hot Chocolate with Fat-Free Milk
(medium, 16 fl oz)
310 calories
6 g fat
(3.5 g saturated)
47 g sugars

Chocolate Triple Thick Shake
(medium, 21 fl oz)
770 calories
18 g fat
(11 g saturated,
1 g trans)
111 g sugars

The iced coffees at McDonald's come pre-loaded with sugar and "light cream," an industrial concoction that contains chemicals like sodium stearoyl lactylate, datem, and tetra sodium pyrophosphate—not the sort of ingredients you want polluting your joe.

GUILTY PLEASURE

McDouble
390 calories
19 g fat (8 g saturated)
920 mg sodium

This $1 burger may be one of the best-selling burgers in America, but in the pantheon of popular patties, this one is relatively harmless, with just 90 calories more than a regular cheeseburger.

OLIVE GARDEN

● Olive Garden's beverage menu is surprisingly mild despite the oversize loads of carbohydrates that come piled on most of the restaurant's plates. The bulk of the cocktails fall within the 200-calorie range, and you're better still if you opt for the meal's wine pairing. Limit yourself to one glass of vino and you'll keep the damage down to 150 calories or so.

2,235

The amount of sodium, in milligrams, in the average plate of pasta from Olive Garden. This represents 93 percent of your recommended daily intake.

Drink This
Wild Berry Bellini

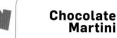

160 calories

You won't find an ice-blended cocktail with fewer calories at any bar or restaurant in the country. Plus, sparkling wine—used to make this riff on a classic Italian drink—has been found to have the same heart-healthy polyphenols found in red wine. Cheers to that!

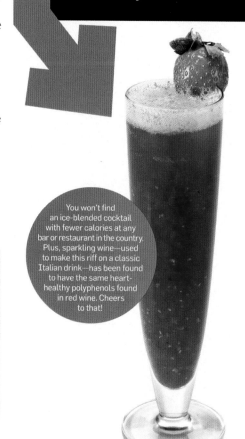

Other Picks

Chocolate Martini
260 calories

Caffe Mocha
180 calories

Sicilian Splash
100 calories

350 calories

Not That!

Strawberry-Mango Frozen Margarita

Other Passes

Chocolate Almond Amore

600 calories

Frozen Cappuccino

320 calories

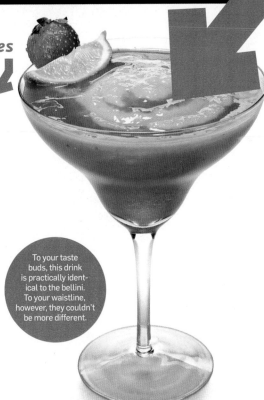

To your taste buds, this drink is practically identical to the bellini. To your waistline, however, they couldn't be more different.

Cream Soda

200 calories

WEAPON OF MASS DESTRUCTION
Chicken and Shrimp Carbonara

1,440 calories
88 g fat
(38 g saturated)
300 mg sodium

On their own, chicken and shrimp are among the world's leanest proteins. Combined in this pasta dish, they deliver two days' worth of saturated fat and as much salt as you'd find in 8 medium orders of McDonald's French fries. The 440-calorie Linguine all Marinara is the best pasta on the menu.

KILLER APP

Caprese Flatbread

600 calories
33 g fat
(10.5 g saturated)
1,520 mg sodium

A cocktail and a flatbread offer a lighter, more sophisticated spin on beer and pizza. Split this with a couple friends after work and you'll take in only 200 calories apiece, which is about half as much as you'd consume if you ordered from the choose-three Sampler Italiano.

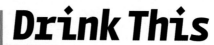

OUTBACK STEAKHOUSE

C-	D+
Drink Report Card	Food Report Card

Drink This

BV Coastal Pinot Noir

California

150 calories

● Thanks to Outback for finally, after years of silence, giving up the nutritional info on their food and beverages. We now know what they were hiding: 2,000-calorie slabs of ribs, 1,800-calorie racks of lamb, 600-calorie sweet potatoes, and a beverage menu with only two truly healthy options on it: wine and coffee. Proceed with caution.

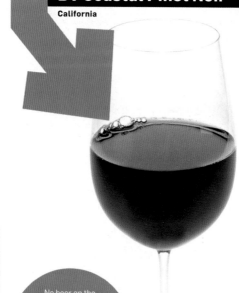

No beer on the planet can rival red wine's antioxidant muscle, and in terms of flavor, pinot noir is among the most versatile. It pairs exceptionally well with Outback-style cuisine: steak, fish, and heavy pastas.

Other Picks

The Gold Coast 'Rita'
170 calories

Captain's Mai Tai
210 calories

Heineken
140 calories

KILLER APP

Seared Ahi Tuna
331 calories
21 g fat
(2.5 g saturated)

Don't fall victim to the lineup of bready, fried appetizers at Outback. Both the Bloomin Onion and the Aussie Cheese Fries will shackle your table with more than 1,500 calories, mostly from refined carbs and residual oil from the deep fryer. Instead, aim to start your meal with a dose of protein and healthy fat. Both encourage satiety, and both are found in abundance in this tasty tuna app.

180 calories

Not That!
Newcastle Brown Ale

ON TAP

Coopers Premium Lager:
180 calories

Coopers Sparkling Ale:
180 calories

James Boag's Premium Lager:
180 calories

Samuel Adams Boston Lager:
180 calories

Budweiser:
144 calories

Corona Extra:
150 calories

Foster's Lager:
150 calories

Amstel Light:
100 calories

Bud Light:
100 calories

Budweiser Select:
99 calories

Coors Light:
100 calories

Corona Light:
100 calories

Michelob ULTRA:
100 calories

Other Passes

Top Shelf Patron Margarita
280 calories

New South Wales Sangria
310 calories

Samuel Adams Boston Lager
180 calories

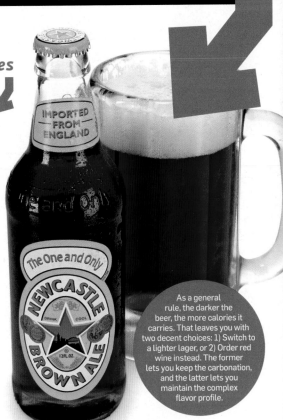

As a general rule, the darker the beer, the more calories it carries. That leaves you with two decent choices: 1) Switch to a lighter lager, or 2) Order red wine instead. The former lets you keep the carbonation, and the latter lets you maintain the complex flavor profile.

PANERA BREAD

● The reason Panera scores better than the more dedicated coffee shops is that it keeps the number of egregious calorie bombs to a minimum. It serves the normal options—the lattes and cappuccinos—along with a daily flavored coffee at most locations. One thing the chain might consider, though, is introducing a sugar-free syrup to accompany the flavored espresso drinks. Oh, that and eliminating the "largo"-size frozen drinks altogether.

Drink This

Chai Tea Latte

(10 fl oz)

200 calories
4.5 g fat
(2.5 g saturated)
32 g sugars

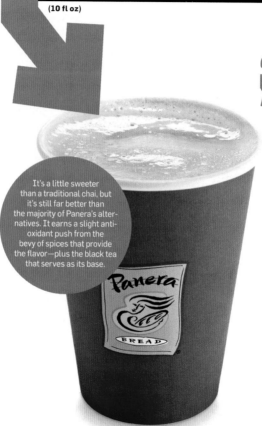

It's a little sweeter than a traditional chai, but it's still far better than the majority of Panera's alternatives. It earns a slight antioxidant push from the bevy of spices that provide the flavor—plus the black tea that serves as its base.

Other Picks

Strawberry Smoothie
(largo, 21.5 fl oz)
290 calories
1.5 g fat
(0.5 g saturated)
48 g sugars

Raspberry Tea
(regular, 20 fl oz)
190 calories
0 g fat
51 g sugars

Frozen Lemonade
(grande, 16 fl oz)
90 calories
0 g fat
22 g sugars

FOOD COURT

THE CRIME
Large Frozen Mocha
(670 calories,
19 g saturated fat)

THE PUNISHMENT
Walk 7.8 miles

420 calories
18 g fat (12 g saturated, 0.5 g trans)
49 g sugars

Not That!

Caramel Latte

(11.5 fl oz)

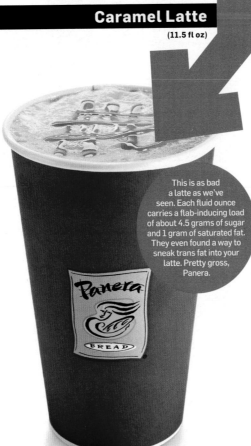

This is as bad a latte as we've seen. Each fluid ounce carries a flab-inducing load of about 4.5 grams of sugar and 1 gram of saturated fat. They even found a way to sneak trans fat into your latte. Pretty gross, Panera.

Other Passes

Frozen Caramel
(largo, 20 fl oz)
710 calories
30 g fat
(17 g saturated)
89 g sugars

Fruit Punch
(regular, 20 fl oz)
260 calories
0 g fat
68 g sugars

Jones Soda Green Apple
(1 bottle, 12.5 fl oz)
180 calories
0 g fat
43 g sugars

BEVERAGE MYTH

Decaffeinated coffee is caffeine free.

Caffeine occurs naturally in coffee beans, and removing it is a challenge akin to stripping the potassium from a banana. Of the 10 cups tested by Florida researchers, only one was truly caffeine free, and it was an instant brand. The other joes had roughly a tenth of that found in regular coffee.

RED LOBSTER

● Red Lobster may be one of our favorite places to eat in America, but it's far from the best place to drink. Alongside the long list of hyper-sweetened coladas, daiquiris, and mudslides is a slew of nearly-as-troublesome virgin libations. Don't ruin a dinner of lean, tasty seafood with a single bad beverage decision.

For 700 calories, you can have

ALL THIS

Seafood Stuffed Flounder, a ½ Pound of North Pacific Crab Legs, a Baked Potato with Sour Cream, and a Cup of Bayou Seafood Gumbo

OR

THAT

A Strawberry Lobsterita

Drink This

Berry Mango Virgin Daiquiri

nonalcoholic

210 calories
0 g fat
52 g carbs

Drink this along with a heavy dose of seafood protein so that your body is better able to fight the tide of incoming glucose. Oh, and be sure to limit yourself to just one. Nonalcoholic and calorie-free are two very different things.

Other Picks

Malibu Hurricane

200 calories
0 g fat
36 g carbs

Sail Away Sunset Strawberry Smoothie

250 calories
6 g fat
(4 g saturated)
47 g carbs

Bailey's and Coffee

180 calories
8 g fat
(5 g saturated)
15 g carbs

340 calories
9 g fat
(6 g saturated)
63 g carbs

Not That!

Berry Strawberry Banana Sail Away Smoothie

nonalcoholic

Other Passes

Bahama Mama

350 calories
0 g fat
51 g carbs

Virgin Strawberry Margarita

340 calories
0 g fat
85 g carbs

Mudslide

520 calories
21 g fat
(13 g saturated)
52 g carbs

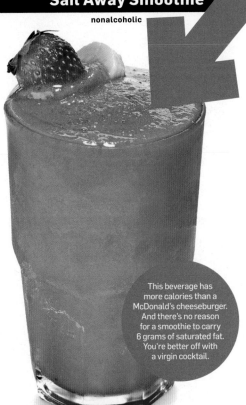

This beverage has more calories than a McDonald's cheeseburger. And there's no reason for a smoothie to carry 6 grams of saturated fat. You're better off with a virgin cocktail.

COCKTAIL DECODER
(Listed best to worst)

SCREWDRIVER: You won't find anything better than this 100-calorie vodka-OJ combo.

CARAMEL APPLETINI: Vodka, apple puckers, and caramel, and yet it packs just 160 calories.

BAHAMA MAMA: Tropical fruit "flavors" mixed with two types of rum. More calories than 7 cooked lobsters.

SUNSET PASSION COLADA: Strawberry-topped piña colada with about half as many calories as the Alotta Colada.

ALOTTA COLADA: A super-size piña colada packing more calories (700) than a Whopper.

TRADITIONAL LOBSTERITA: With 900 calories, the worst cocktail in America.

KILLER APP

Chilled Jumbo Shrimp Cocktail

120 calories
1 g fat (0 g saturated)
590 mg sodium

Among its many merits, shrimp is loaded with vitamin D, and a study of 3,000 men ages 40 to 79 confirmed that those with higher levels of this vitamin performed better on mental-agility tests.

85

TGI FRIDAY'S

D+
Drink Report Card

D−
Food Report Card

● Friday's seems to fancy itself as much a bar as it does a restaurant, which could be a good thing, since its food is pretty unhealthy. But unfortunately, Friday's has compiled an impressively long list of sugary cocktails and beers and has little to offer in the form of low-calorie, high-nutrient, booze-free beverages.

Drink This
Top Shelf Mojito

220 calories

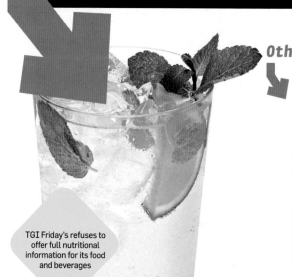

TGI Friday's refuses to offer full nutritional information for its food and beverages

The surge in the mojito's popularity over the past decade means that what was once an obscure Cuban cocktail is now one of the lightest libations you'll find on any restaurant menu.

Other Picks

Ultimate Margarita Frozen
190 calories

Ultimate Mango Mai Tai
290 calories

Strawberry Lemonade Slush
(nonalcoholic)
240 calories

KILLER APP

Zen Chicken Pot Stickers
370 calories

Friday's invented the potato skin, and its greasy claim-to-fame is the 2,270-calorie anchor to a horrific appetizer menu. These tasty pan-fried Asian dumplings are a welcome beacon of health in an otherwise dark and troubling world. They go great with a cocktail, so grab a mojito and a friend and have at it. Just be sure to skip the rest of dinner.

400 calories

Not That!

Ultimate Margarita Pomegranate

ON TAP

Newcastle Brown Ale: 180 calories

Blue Moon: 164 calories

Killian's Irish Red: 162 calories

Bass Ale: 156 calories

Corona Extra: 148 calories

Budweiser: 144 calories

Rolling Rock: 132 calories

Michelob Light: 123 calories

Corona Light: 105 calories

Heineken Premium Light: 99 calories

Amstel Light: 95 calories

Other Passes

Electric Lemonade
290 calories

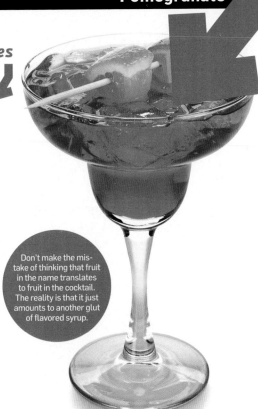

Hawaii Volcano
380 calories

Don't make the mistake of thinking that fruit in the name translates to fruit in the cocktail. The reality is that it just amounts to another glut of flavored syrup.

Cherry Limeade Slush
510 calories

FOOD COURT

THE CRIME
Ultimate Strawberry Daiquiri
(490 calories)

THE PUNISHMENT
2 hours chopping wood

UNO CHICAGO GRILL

● Uno didn't earn its grade through an extensive selection of extremely nutritious options, but more so from a list of not-too-awful indulgences. Its smoothies all start with fatfree yogurt and its sweetened slushes are properly proportioned. If it applied the same restraint to the food menu, it'd be a truly healthy restaurant.

Drink This
Chocolate Monkey
nonalcoholic

260 calories
6 g fat
(0 g saturated)
45 g sugars

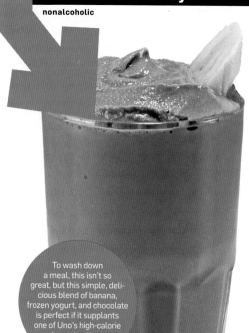

To wash down a meal, this isn't so great, but this simple, delicious blend of banana, frozen yogurt, and chocolate is perfect if it supplants one of Uno's high-calorie dessert options.

Other Picks

Fresh Lemon Drop Martini
230 calories

House Chardonnay
110 calories

Samuel Adams Light
(bottle, 12 fl oz)
124 calories

480 calories
14 g fat
(4.5 g saturated,
2.5 g trans)
46 g sugars

Not That!

Chocolate Cookie Freezer

nonalcoholic

Other Passes

Wildberry Lemonade
310 calories

Chateau Ste. Michelle Riesling
180 calories

Uno Amber Ale
(14 fl oz)
220 calories

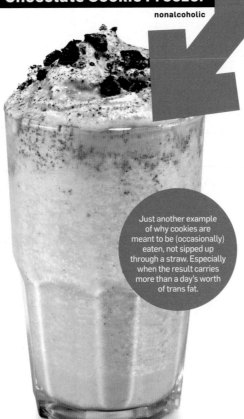

Just another example of why cookies are meant to be (occasionally) eaten, not sipped up through a straw. Especially when the result carries more than a day's worth of trans fat.

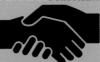

PERFECT PARTNER

Steak on a Stick with Roasted Seasonal Vegetables

390 calories
14.5 g fat
(4 g saturated)
1,500 mg sodium

Navigating Uno's menu can be like walking blindfolded through a minefield. Once you tack on sides and Uno's nefarious bread-sticks, few of the plates come served with less than 1,000 calories. This new menu addition, however, bucks the trend, providing plenty of lean protein and a good array of vegetable-driven nutrients for a meager caloric sum.

FOOD COURT

THE CRIME
Chicago Classic Individual Deep Dish Pizza
(2,310 calories)

THE PUNISHMENT
Tread water for 8 hours

Chapter

3

Drink This, Not That!

SOFT DRINKS

As kids growing up in Pennsylvania's Lehigh Valley, my brother and I often spent autumns visiting nearby farms. We'd pick out our pumpkins from the pumpkin patch, drink hot cider from a cart, and walk through a maze carved from neat, symmetrical, seemingly endless rows of corn. Around Halloween, high school kids would make extra cash dressing up as zombies and helping to turn those corn mazes into scary theme parks.

CHAPTER 3

Today, even those of us who live in the city, in the desert, or in the tropics can walk through scary corn mazes all year long. Except those long, endless rows of horror aren't at your local farm. They're at your local supermarket. Because when you walk down the soda aisle, that's exactly what you're seeing: endless rows of liquid corn.

And that liquid corn can do a lot more damage to your body than fake zombies can.

Corn—refined, reconfigured, and liquefied—is the basic building material of almost all soft drinks sold in America today. In fact, Americans drink an average of 200 calories a day in high-fructose corn syrup, or HFCS, alone—that's enough to pack on nearly 21 pounds of extra weight in a year. (And one in five of us drink a whopping 505 HFCS calories daily!) That makes HFCS almost as ubiquitous as another invention from 1975, Angelina Jolie. (Also invented around 1975: 50 Cent, David Beckham, Chelsea Handler, and the little push-through tabs on the top of beer cans.)

But the past 35 years haven't been as good to most Americans as they've been to Angelina. Since the time food marketers began adding HFCS to our food and beverages, America's obesity rate has doubled; the health condition most directly tied to obesity—diabetes—eats up one in five of our health care dollars, and obesity may soon surpass tobacco as the number one cause of death. (Makes the dual threats of paparazzi and Jennifer Aniston pale in comparison, huh?) The average American man now consumes about 7 percent more calories a day than in the 1970s; the average woman a whopping 22 percent more.

And while HFCS is everywhere (check your salad dressing, your wheat bread, even your ketchup!), soda and other sweetened beverages are our number one sources of it.

Now, you may think that one or two cans of soda a day isn't that big a deal. It's not like other terrible habits, like drugs, alcohol, cigarettes, or Irish step dancing. But what if I told you that by kicking the soda habit, you could dramatically change not only your diet, but your entire life? Don't believe me? Consider this:

1. Drink less soda, lose weight fast.
Researchers say you can measure a person's risk of obesity by measuring his or her soda intake. Versus people who don't drink sweetened sodas, here's what your daily intake means:

½ can =
26 percent increased risk of being overweight or obese

½ to 1 can =
30.4 percent increased risk

1 to 2 cans =
32.8 percent increased risk

More than 2 cans =
47.2 percent increased risk

That's a pretty remarkable set of stats. You don't have to guzzle Double Gulps from the 7-Eleven to put yourself at risk, you just need to indulge in one or two cans a day. Wow. And because HFCS is so cheap, food marketers keep making serving sizes bigger (even the "small" at most movie theaters is enough to drown a raccoon). That means we're drinking more than ever and don't even realize it: In the 1950s, the average person drank 11 gallons of soda a year. By the mid-2000s, we were drinking 46 gallons a year. A Center for Science in the Public Interest report contained this shocking sentence: "Carbonated soft drinks are the single biggest source of calories in the American diet."

2. Drink less soda, eat smarter automatically. The problem with soda isn't just what's going into our bellies; it's what's not going into our bellies as well. Researchers at Purdue University found that regular soda drinkers consumed 9 percent fewer calories from fresh vegetables and 62 percent fewer calories from fresh fruit. (They ate fewer canned and frozen fruits and vegetables as well.)

3. Drink less soda, make more money. Wait, what? That's crazy. Except that it's not: Those same researchers at

Purdue found that people who don't drink soda have average incomes of $40,300. Regular soda drinkers? Just $35,640. Since employers tend to pay slimmer employees better—because they're viewed as more competent, disciplined, and in control—it's probable that over the long haul, soda can damage your bank account and your career. So tossing out the soda can is like giving yourself a 10 percent raise—without working harder!

4. Drink less soda, lose your beer belly. A 2009 study from the University of California found that fructose can cause your body to build new fat cells around the heart, liver, and digestive organs. When people were given high quantities of calories in either fructose or glucose, both groups gained weight. But the fructose group gained their new fat around their internal organs. That's the "hard beer belly" fat known as visceral fat, and it's far more harmful to your health than the flab that collects in your love handles (known as "subcutaneous" fat).

5. Drink less soda, lower your risk of heart attack. Visceral fat around your internal organs unleashes a group of compounds within your body that causes inflammation and an increase in triglycerides and LDL cholesterol—the bad stuff that leads to heart disease and stroke.

6. Drink less soda, feel less hungry. When researchers from Purdue gave people 450 calories to consume from either jelly beans or soda, the candy eaters took in no more total calories over the course of the day than usual. The soda swiggers, however, downed 17 percent more calories each day. Liquid calories from sugar appear to have an opposite effect on satiety, in essence making you hungrier as you drink. As a result, the more soda calories you guzzle, the more food calories you crave. Crazy, right?

BOTTOM LINE

Cutting down on soda calories—and calories from other sweetened beverages like iced teas—is the fastest, easiest way to lose weight, improve your health, and even boost your income. In the following pages, we'll show you how to do just that.

Now, aren't you glad you bought this book?

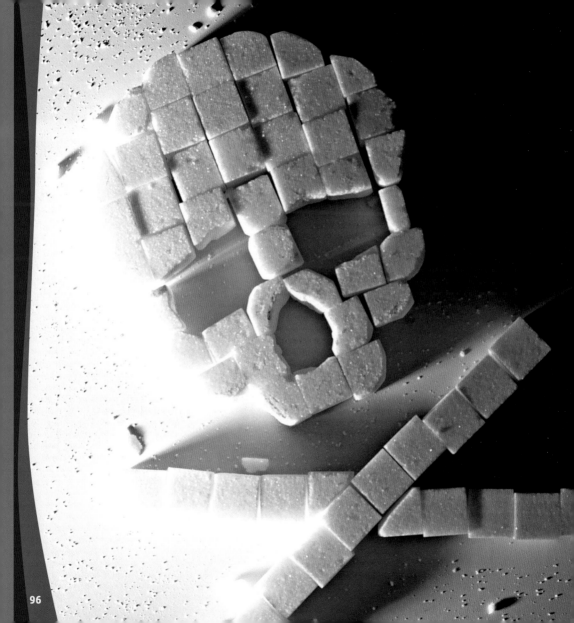

Public Enemy #1

Forget Dillinger, Dahmer, and Manson—America's deadliest criminal is lurking in your pantry

If sugar were a drug, then we'd be a nation of junkies. According to the National Health and Nutrition Examination Survey, Americans consume 22 teaspoons of added sugar a day, a quantity that saddles each one of us with 330 unnecessary calories. And what's the number one source of all that surreptitious sweetness? Yup, you guessed it: beverages. Not just soft drinks, but teas, "enhanced" waters, and so-called juice drinks.

The problem isn't just that sugar has been directly linked to so many deadly diseases—cancer, cardiovascular disease, diabetes—but that sugar offers us absolutely nothing in return for its sticky caloric surge. Therein lies the central pitfall of our drinking problem: Whereas most foods arrive on your plate swimming in a vast array of macro and micronutrients—protein, fat, fiber, calcium, folate, and so on—which help keep our bellies full and our bodies functioning at peak levels, the overwhelming majority of beverages owe their entire caloric content to the dreaded white powder.

Sugar bears the mask of many monikers—high-fructose corn syrup, evaporated cane juice, fructose, sucrose—but regardless of the form and name it takes, its impact on our bodies is devastating. Consider what happens to our systems when we drink, say, a can of Coke:

Within minutes, your body is hit with 8 teaspoons of sugar, a quantity that sets off a deleterious chain reaction of biochemical responses. First, your blood sugar levels spike dramatically, forcing your pancreas to secrete insulin in an attempt to lower those levels. Your body works rapidly to convert the sugar into fuel, but with so much sugar released into the bloodstream so quickly, you have more fuel than you need; the excess sugar that your body can't use immediately is then turned into fat. Next, your body begins to release dopamine, the same feel-good neurotransmitter kicked into gear by drugs like marijuana and heroin. It's this step that keeps us coming back for more. All is great for a few moments, but when your body has finally chewed through all of that sugar, blood glucose levels will fall rapidly, bringing about the full scale sugar crash. The end result: Less energy, more fat. The worst of all worlds.

The solution, of course, is to cut added sugar out of your life wherever possible, starting with beverages. In order to reduce the risk of heart disease, cancer, diabetes, and obesity, the American Heart Association recommends that women limit their added sugar intake to 100 calories and men to 150 calories. The easiest move is to trade regular soft drinks for diet and rely on sugar-free products wherever possible (for more on the best and worst sugar substitutes, read "The Truth About Alternative Sweeteners" on page 101), but really, the goal is to crowd sweeteners—real and artificial—out of your diet by loading up on fresh fruits and vegetables and turning to that old reliable friend of ours: water.

The Truth About
High-Fructose Corn Syrup

In 1970, there was about half a pound of high-fructose corn syrup produced for every person in the United States. By the time we entered the new millennium, that number had escalated to more than 60 pounds. That means that every year each of us is responsible for consuming the weight of a Labrador retriever in the form of highly processed, corn-derived sugar, which will enter our bodies disguised in hundreds of different vessels: canned fruits and vegetables, pasta sauces, frozen dinners, ice creams, candies, crackers, yogurts, puddings, teas, juices, sodas, and any number of other ubiquitous and shelf-stable supermarket products.

This becomes especially concerning when you hear nutritional pundits discussing escalating obesity rates and HFCS in the same breath. Plenty of money and time has been invested in researching corn sweeteners in hopes of pegging them as the leading cause of weight gain. Scientists are right to be looking, too—the obesity rate has more than doubled since HFCS made it onto the menu. Problem is, nobody's discovered the invisible thread linking HFCS to weight gain, and those who've come closest were really just looking at fructose, which is demonstrably different from HFCS. So what's a shopper to think? Here's everything you need to know.

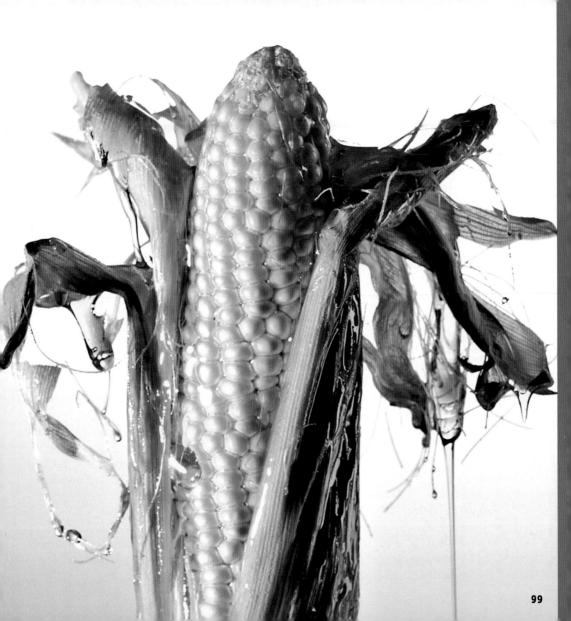

High-fructose corn syrup is essentially identical to regular table sugar.

Their biggest difference boils down to the ratio of fructose to glucose, the two sugar molecules that comprise both sweeteners. Table sugar, or sucrose, consists of a 50-50 blend of fructose to glucose. HFCS, on the other hand, comes primarily in two forms: One combines fructose and glucose in a ratio of 42-58, and the other blends the two in a ratio of 55-45. That makes them both very close to sucrose. It also puts them in the same ballpark as other common sweeteners such as honey and fruit juice concentrates. What's more, all forms of sugar have exactly 4 calories per gram, which means you can't cut your energy intake by switching to a better sugar.

High-fructose corn syrup is a dream come true for the package foods industry.

While HFCS might not be technically worse for our bodies than sugar, it is more likely to find its way into our diets. For many years, sugar posed a few problems for packaged food producers. Not only was it relatively expensive, but it has a short shelf life and, because of its granular texture, proved difficult to incorporate into certain products. Then some scientists figured out what to do with all that extra corn our farmers were growing and along came HFCS to solve all of these problems. Now producers were armed with a cheap, shelf-stable liquid that could be incorporated seamlessly into tens of thousands of packaged goods. Without getting too political here, the United States Farm Bill is really at the heart of this problem. The bill subsidizes the production of more corn than this country needs, driving down the price of HFCS and providing us with a seemingly endless supply of syrupy sweetener that can be used to increase the palatability of foods that traditionally were never meant to be sweetened. (Think Grandma was tossing sugar into her whole wheat bread loaves back in the '40s?) The worst part? Americans are hit with the cost of sky-high health insurance as a result of the millions fighting type 2 diabetes and other chronic diseases exacerbated by our consumption of HFCS and other sugars. The National Diabetes Economic Barometer study found that diabetes alone cost the United States $217 billion in 2007. So we pay on the front end to subsidize the industrial-scale production of corn sweeteners and then again on the back end when all that superfluous sweetness in our food supply makes us sick.

There is no such thing as "healthy" sugar.

Sugar is more than just a source of empty calories, it's a fierce and unforgiving calorie vacuum, sucking up our hard-earned daily allotment and leaving nothing in return. Sugar is responsible for little else beyond providing a bit of quick-burning energy, the kind that throws your blood sugar into turmoil as it moves from short-term storage in your stomach to long-term storage as flab on your belly. Table sugar and HFCS are both equally guilty of this. Higher-end sweeteners such as honey and maple syrup do come bundled with a smattering of nutrients, but it's not really enough to justify the caloric price tag. You don't eat sugar for sustenance; you eat for pleasure.

The Truth About
Alternative
Sweeteners

Once upon a time, sugar was sugar, and when a host offered you coffee or tea, they served it alongside a small glass bowl or porcelain jar. The spoon protruding from the top led straight down to a mound of pure, granulated table sugar. That was your only option for sweetening a beverage. Today you order tea and it comes with a plastic box bulging with a rainbow of options that represent decades of research and advancement distilled down into tiny paper packages. There are pinks, blues, browns, and whites—some with calories and some without. Picking one packet over another can make a profound statement about your health values: I won't be swayed by the newest fad, or I prefer to risk cancer than look bad in a bathing suit.

The problem is the statement we're making isn't always clear. The sweeteners are rolling out so fast that we can hardly keep up with which ones are safe and which ones cause us to grow new appendages. In the supermarket, they're usually buried under an avalanche of complex-sounding ingredients that you need a microscope and a doctorate degree just to decipher. The whole thing is more confusing than health care reform.

To help straighten you out, we've put together a list of the most prevalent alternative sweeteners. These are the ones that tend to have big corporate sponsors spending millions of dollars to convince you that theirs is the safest and tastiest of all the sweeteners. Some are indeed safe, but others should be avoided at all costs. Read on to find which is which.

Acesulfame Potassium
(Or Acesulfame-K, Ace K)

In 2003, the FDA approved this calorie-free artificial sweetener for use in everything outside of meat and poultry. It's 200 times sweeter than sugar and now appears in more than 5,000 foods and drinks. But rarely will you see it on its own. Like other artificial sweeteners, ace K delivers a bitter aftertaste. That's why it almost always appears alongside aspartame or sucralose, the idea being that sweeteners

in tandem will balance each other and mask any off flavors.

RISK ASSESSMENT:
Limit consumption. Many health and industry insiders question the FDA's judgment in approving acesulfame-K. Animal studies have linked it to lung and breast tumors, and large doses have caused thyroid problems in rats, rabbits, and dogs. But so far, these adverse effects have yet to be borne out in human studies.

FOUND IN:
Powerade Zero, Coca-Cola Zero, Diet Snapple Tea, Sugar Free Rockstar, Sugar Free Red Bull, Diet Ocean Spray Cranberry Grape, Diet V8 Splash, Arizona Diet Green Tea with Ginseng

Agave Nectar

This sweetener is culled from Mexico's cactuslike blue agave, the same wonder plant that gives us tequila. When bottlers use it to sweeten beverages, they do so with the implied or stated claim that it's a natural alternative to traditional sweeteners. Unfortunately, this isn't entirely true. Blue agave itself is natural, but the sugars aren't readily available in the plant's raw form. To draw them out, processors

use acids or enzymes to break down inulin fibers, and it's a technical process that wasn't applied to agave until sometime during the '90s. The result is sweeter than sugar and delivers about 60 calories per tablespoon.

RISK ASSESSMENT:

Safe for consumption. The research is limited on this relatively new sweetener, but it's probably best to think of it as just another form of sugar. The upside is that it's sweeter than sucrose, so you can generally get by using less. It also has an impressively low glycemic index, so unlike table sugar, it has a mild effect on your blood sugar. But agave nectar contains as much as 90 percent fructose, and studies on the monosaccharide have shown it to increase triglyceride levels and pad your liver with visceral fat. Plus an analysis published by the *Journal of the American Dietetic Association* found that, in terms of antioxidants, agave syrup is far closer to refined sugar or corn syrup than it is to legitimate natural sweeteners like molasses, maple syrup, or honey.

FOUND IN:

Honest Tea Agave Mate, Numi Earl Grey Organic Puerh Black Tea, Oogavé Cola, Lakewood Light Organic Lemonade, Bossa Nova Acai Juice

Aspartame

Aspartame has been the focal point of the most ardent anti-artificial-sweetener campaigns, yet still it maintains a supermarket stronghold with some 6,000 products to its credit. The reason? It's cheap, 180 times sweeter than sugar, and virtually calorie free. (It actually has 4 calories per gram, but you'd have to drink nearly a six-pack to reach that level.) It's found in the vast majority of diet soft drinks as well as teas and juices, and it's sold under the brand names NutraSweet and Equal. Although many beverage makers are starting to move toward other artificial sweeteners, it's unlikely that we'll see the end of aspartame anytime soon—it has, after all, enjoyed more than three decades as a completely legal food additive.

RISK ASSESSMENT:

Limit consumption. Thousands of aspartame-related complaints have been submitted to the FDA and the Department of Health and Human Services for symptoms such as headaches, dizziness, diarrhea, memory loss, and mood changes, and the Center for Science in the Public Interest recommends that children avoid aspartame-sweetened beverages. The FDA upholds the sweetener's safety, but the studies aren't always so convincing. Some find it to be harmless, while others implicate it in brain cancer, lymphoma, and leukemia.

Safe for consumption. Considering it far superior to aspartame, the Center for Science in the Public Interest has declared neotame fit for consumption. The only other artificial sweetener to earn the center's support is sucralose.

Clabber Girl Sugar Replacer, Domino Pure D'Lite, and *Hostess 100-Calorie Packs*

NutraSweet, Equal, Diet Snapple Peach Tea, Sugar Free Red Bull, Diet Pepsi, Diet Sunkist, Schweppes Diet Ginger Ale, Diet Dr. Pepper, Sprite Zero

Saccharin

The oldest artificial sweetener was discovered in 1879 and is 300 to 500 times sweeter than sugar. Between 1977 and 2000, the FDA mandated that products made with saccharin carry a warning label educating consumers about the sweetener's link to cancer. Today, however, saccharin can be legally buried in the list of ingredients. Thankfully, the discovery of safer sweeteners has helped to nudge it out of many recipes, but it's still not completely phased out.

Neotame

Chemically, neotame is similar to aspartame, and in fact both chemicals are produced by NutraSweet. The difference is that neotame is stable enough to withstand high cooking temperatures, and it's about 40 times stronger, which makes it by far the most powerful of the noncaloric sweeteners. In fact, you would need about 4,000 teaspoons of sugar to equal the sweetening power of a ½ teaspoon of neotame. The FDA approved it in 2002, and its popularity has been growing steadily since.

Avoid entirely. The FDA's warning label took effect after the sweetener was linked to bladder tumors in rats, and other studies linked it to cancers of the ovaries, bladder, and skin.

This was repealed after the FDA decided that the studies posed no reasonable threat to humans. In other words, saccharin will be tolerated unless somebody proves beyond a doubt that it causes cancer in humans. (Shouldn't it work the other way around—that we only allow something into the food supply once it's been proven safe?) Regardless, one recent study funded by Purdue and the National Institutes of Health showed that rats with a saccharin-rich diet gained more weight than those eating real sugar. And with a wide range of safer sweeteners on the market, there's no reason to risk it.

FOUND IN:

Sweet 'N Low, TaB Cola

Stevia

Although it's been around for years, the FDA didn't approve stevia for use in processed foods and beverages until the end of 2008. Now it's the only noncaloric sweetener you'll find that can claim to be directly descended from a plant, or more specifically, a South American shrub called *Stevia rebaudiana*. (The term "stevia" refers to the plant, while the more-refined version of the sweetener is called "rebiana" or "reb A.") It's 100 times sweeter than sugar, and, because of a faint licoricelike aftertaste, it's often blended with real sugar or other artificial sweeteners.

RISK ASSESSMENT:

Limit consumption. Initial rodent studies have shown a potential for fertility problems and DNA damage, which is why the Center for Science in the Public Interest warns consumers to limit their intake until further studies can be conducted. If future testing on humans proves stevia to be safe, then the agency will lift its warning.

FOUND IN:

Truvia, PureVia, Sun Crystals, SoBé Lifewater, Vitamin Water, Sprite Green, Tropicana Trop50

Sucralose

The FDA approved sucralose in 1998 after reviewing more than 110 studies on animals and humans. The noncaloric sweetener's most ardent proponents hail it as a close relative of sugar, and in fact its name is a phonetic reference to sucrose. But really the two are quite different. Sucralose production might begin with sugar, but the two cease to be alike when the molecules are bound with chlorine atoms to create a new substance with 600 times the sweetness of table sugar.

Safe for consumption. As one of the most well-studied food additives, sucralose is largely regarded as the safest of the artificial sweeteners. Plus it was the first to earn an endorsement from the Center for Science in the Public Interest, which tends to be a tough institute to win over. (Neotame is the only other artificial sweetener to earn this distinction.) That being said, some studies indicate that artificial sweeteners of any kind can lead to extra calorie consumption at subsequent meals. The promise of calories with no payoff, the researchers argue, makes your body crave energy. Plus the simple act of training your tongue to desire sweet foods can make you less satisfied with unsweetened foods.

FOUND IN:

Splenda, Hansen's Diet Soda, Pepsi One, Lipton Pure Leaf Diet Lemon, Diet V8 Splash, Lo-Carb Monster Energy, Myoplex Carb Control, Ocean Spray Cranergy Energy Juice Drink, Capri Sun Roarin' Waters, Amp Energy Sugar Free

The Truth About
Diet
Soda

When confronted with the growing tide of calories from sweetened beverages, the first response is, "Why not just drink diet soda?" Well, for a few reasons:

Just because diet soda is low in calories doesn't mean it can't lead to weight gain. It may have only 5 or fewer calories per serving, but emerging research suggests that consuming sugary-tasting beverages—even if they're artificially sweetened—may lead to a high preference for sweetness overall. That means sweeter (and more caloric) cereal, bread, dessert—everything.

There remain some concerns about aspartame, the low-calorie chemical used to give diet sodas their flavor.

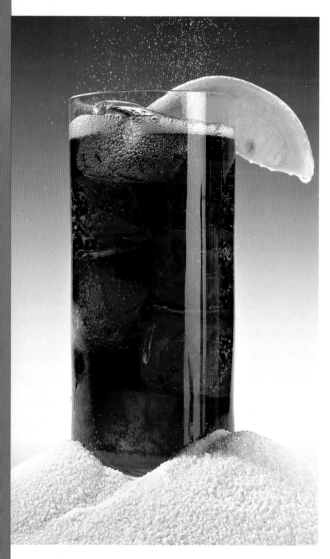

Aspartame is 180 times sweeter than sugar, and some animal research has linked consumption of high amounts of the sweetener to brain tumors and lymphoma in rodents. The FDA maintains that the sweetener is safe, but reported side effects include dizziness, headaches, diarrhea, memory loss, and mood changes.

The diet soda dilemma is more than just a matter of one or two suspect sweeteners. Guzzling these drinks all day long forces out the healthy beverages you need. Diet soda is 100 percent nutrition-free, and again, it's just as important to actively drink the good stuff as it is to avoid that bad stuff. So one diet soda a day is fine, but if you're downing five or six cans, that means you're limiting your intake of healthful beverages, particularly water and tea.

BOTTOM LINE

Diet soda does you no good, and it might just be doing you wrong. The best way to hydrate is by drinking low-calorie, high-nutrient fluids—and avoiding belt-busting beverages like the 20 Worst Drinks in America.

The Anatomy of America's Most Popular Beverages

Discover the secret (and not-so-secret) formulas of the drinks Americans love most

Ever wonder what you're really drinking? The FDA has approved 3,000 food additives, and no doubt more than a few of them are floating around in your favorite beverage. Find out how 10 popular drinks are made, from the healthy and straightforward to the disturbingly scientific.

Cola

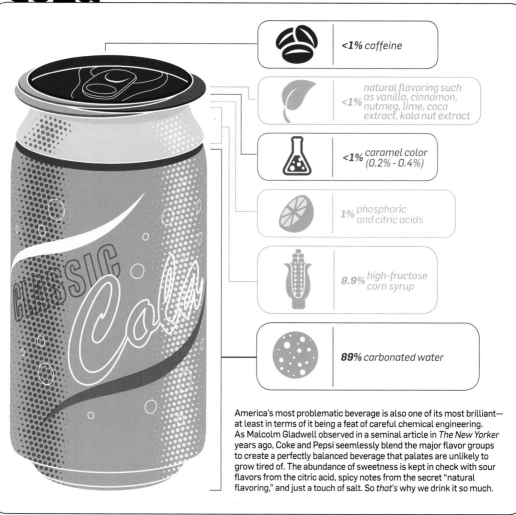

<1% *caffeine*

<1% *natural flavoring such as vanilla, cinnamon, nutmeg, lime, coca extract, kola nut extract*

<1% *caramel color (0.2% - 0.4%)*

1% *phosphoric and citric acids*

8.9% *high-fructose corn syrup*

89% *carbonated water*

America's most problematic beverage is also one of its most brilliant—at least in terms of it being a feat of careful chemical engineering. As Malcolm Gladwell observed in a seminal article in *The New Yorker* years ago, Coke and Pepsi seemlessly blend the major flavor groups to create a perfectly balanced beverage that palates are unlikely to grow tired of. The abundance of sweetness is kept in check with sour flavors from the citric acid, spicy notes from the secret "natural flavoring," and just a touch of salt. So *that's* why we drink it so much.

Beer

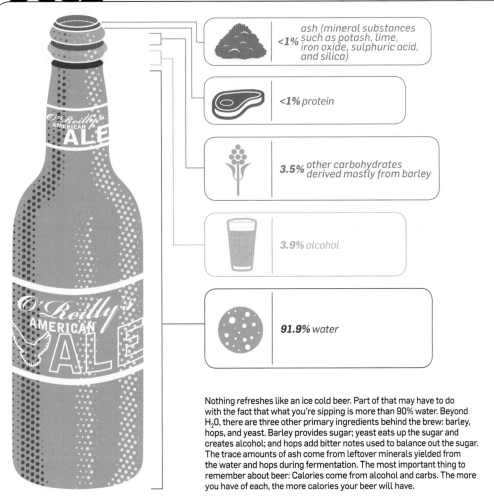

<1% ash (mineral substances such as potash, lime, iron oxide, sulphuric acid, and silica)

<1% protein

3.5% other carbohydrates derived mostly from barley

3.9% alcohol

91.9% water

Nothing refreshes like an ice cold beer. Part of that may have to do with the fact that what you're sipping is more than 90% water. Beyond H_2O, there are three other primary ingredients behind the brew: barley, hops, and yeast. Barley provides sugar; yeast eats up the sugar and creates alcohol; and hops add bitter notes used to balance out the sugar. The trace amounts of ash come from leftover minerals yielded from the water and hops during fermentation. The most important thing to remember about beer: Calories come from alcohol and carbs. The more you have of each, the more calories your beer will have.

Bottled Coffee Drink

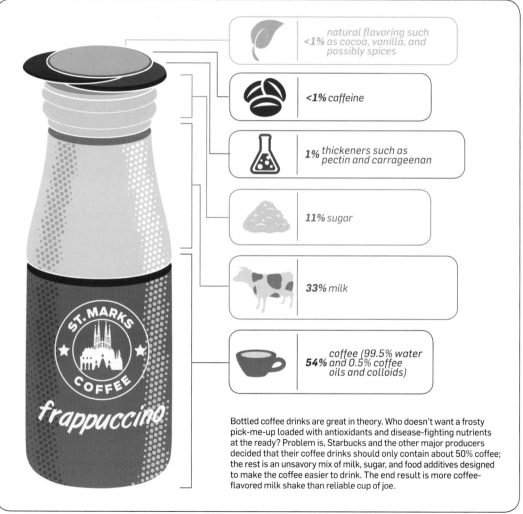

<1% natural flavoring such as cocoa, vanilla, and possibly spices

<1% caffeine

1% thickeners such as pectin and carrageenan

11% sugar

33% milk

54% coffee (99.5% water and 0.5% coffee oils and colloids)

Bottled coffee drinks are great in theory. Who doesn't want a frosty pick-me-up loaded with antioxidants and disease-fighting nutrients at the ready? Problem is, Starbucks and the other major producers decided that their coffee drinks should only contain about 50% coffee; the rest is an unsavory mix of milk, sugar, and food additives designed to make the coffee easier to drink. The end result is more coffee-flavored milk shake than reliable cup of joe.

Cranberry Juice Cocktail

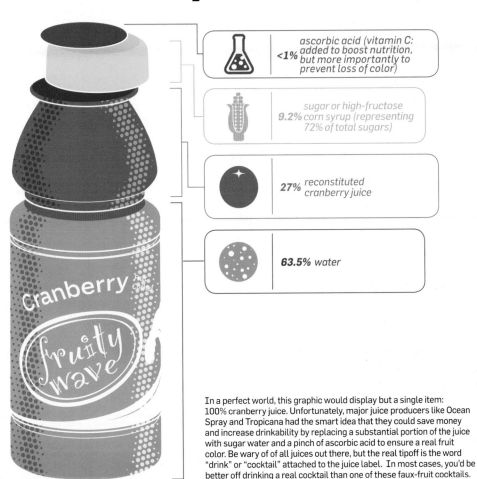

<1% ascorbic acid (vitamin C: added to boost nutrition, but more importantly to prevent loss of color)

9.2% sugar or high-fructose corn syrup (representing 72% of total sugars)

27% reconstituted cranberry juice

63.5% water

In a perfect world, this graphic would display but a single item: 100% cranberry juice. Unfortunately, major juice producers like Ocean Spray and Tropicana had the smart idea that they could save money and increase drinkability by replacing a substantial portion of the juice with sugar water and a pinch of ascorbic acid to ensure a real fruit color. Be wary of of all juices out there, but the real tipoff is the word "drink" or "cocktail" attached to the juice label. In most cases, you'd be better off drinking a real cocktail than one of these faux-fruit cocktails.

Vegetable Juice Blend

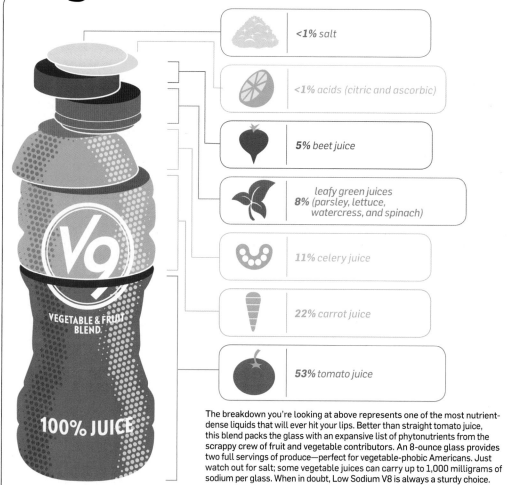

<1% *salt*

<1% *acids (citric and ascorbic)*

5% *beet juice*

8% *leafy green juices (parsley, lettuce, watercress, and spinach)*

11% *celery juice*

22% *carrot juice*

53% *tomato juice*

The breakdown you're looking at above represents one of the most nutrient-dense liquids that will ever hit your lips. Better than straight tomato juice, this blend packs the glass with an expansive list of phytonutrients from the scrappy crew of fruit and vegetable contributors. An 8-ounce glass provides two full servings of produce—perfect for vegetable-phobic Americans. Just watch out for salt; some vegetable juices can carry up to 1,000 milligrams of sodium per glass. When in doubt, Low Sodium V8 is always a sturdy choice.

Lemonade

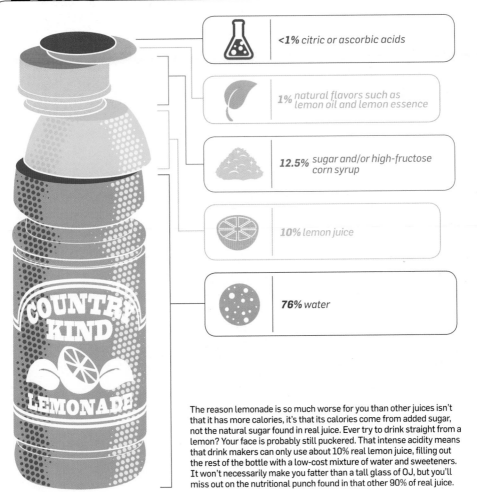

<1% *citric or ascorbic acids*

1% *natural flavors such as lemon oil and lemon essence*

12.5% *sugar and/or high-fructose corn syrup*

10% *lemon juice*

76% *water*

COUNTRY KIND LEMONADE

The reason lemonade is so much worse for you than other juices isn't that it has more calories, it's that its calories come from added sugar, not the natural sugar found in real juice. Ever try to drink straight from a lemon? Your face is probably still puckered. That intense acidity means that drink makers can only use about 10% real lemon juice, filling out the rest of the bottle with a low-cost mixture of water and sweeteners. It won't necessarily make you fatter than a tall glass of OJ, but you'll miss out on the nutritional punch found in that other 90% of real juice.

Energy Drink

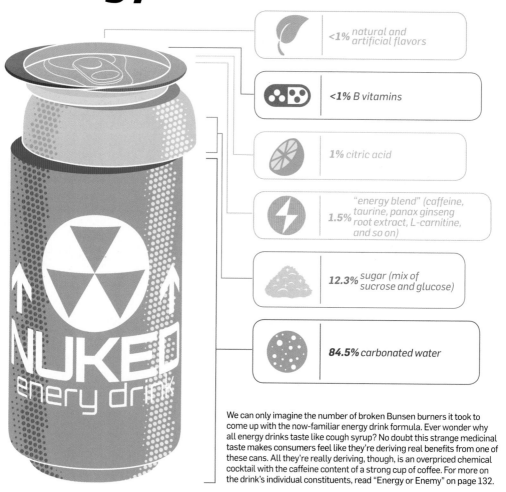

<1% *natural and artificial flavors*

<1% *B vitamins*

1% *citric acid*

1.5% *"energy blend" (caffeine, taurine, panax ginseng root extract, L-carnitine, and so on)*

12.3% *sugar (mix of sucrose and glucose)*

84.5% *carbonated water*

NUKED
enery drink

We can only imagine the number of broken Bunsen burners it took to come up with the now-familiar energy drink formula. Ever wonder why all energy drinks taste like cough syrup? No doubt this strange medicinal taste makes consumers feel like they're deriving real benefits from one of these cans. All they're really deriving, though, is an overpriced chemical cocktail with the caffeine content of a strong cup of coffee. For more on the drink's individual constituents, read "Energy or Enemy" on page 132.

Flavored Iced Tea

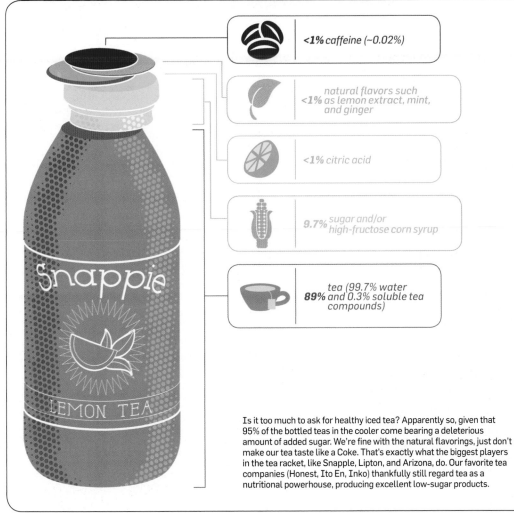

<1% *caffeine (~0.02%)*

<1% *natural flavors such as lemon extract, mint, and ginger*

<1% *citric acid*

9.7% *sugar and/or high-fructose corn syrup*

89% *tea (99.7% water and 0.3% soluble tea compounds)*

Is it too much to ask for healthy iced tea? Apparently so, given that 95% of the bottled teas in the cooler come bearing a deleterious amount of added sugar. We're fine with the natural flavorings, just don't make our tea taste like a Coke. That's exactly what the biggest players in the tea racket, like Snapple, Lipton, and Arizona, do. Our favorite tea companies (Honest, Ito En, Inko) thankfully still regard tea as a nutritional powerhouse, producing excellent low-sugar products.

Vitamin-Enhanced Water

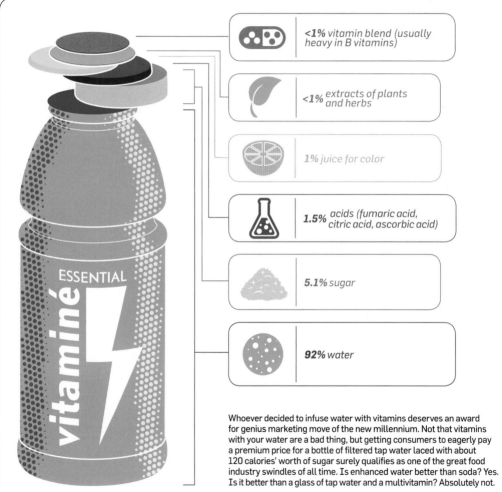

<1% *vitamin blend (usually heavy in B vitamins)*

<1% *extracts of plants and herbs*

1% *juice for color*

1.5% *acids (fumaric acid, citric acid, ascorbic acid)*

5.1% *sugar*

92% *water*

ESSENTIAL
vitaminé

Whoever decided to infuse water with vitamins deserves an award for genius marketing move of the new millennium. Not that vitamins with your water are a bad thing, but getting consumers to eagerly pay a premium price for a bottle of filtered tap water laced with about 120 calories' worth of sugar surely qualifies as one of the great food industry swindles of all time. Is enhanced water better than soda? Yes. Is it better than a glass of tap water and a multivitamin? Absolutely not.

Shelf-stable
Chocolate "Milk" Drink

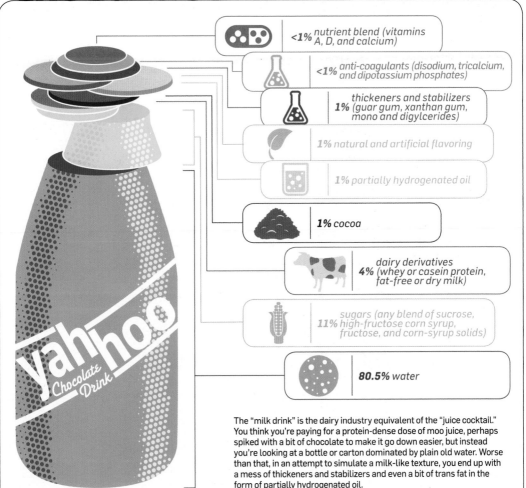

<1% nutrient blend (vitamins A, D, and calcium)

<1% anti-coagulants (disodium, tricalcium, and dipotassium phosphates)

1% thickeners and stabilizers (guar gum, xanthan gum, mono and digylcerides)

1% natural and artificial flavoring

1% partially hydrogenated oil

1% cocoa

4% dairy derivatives (whey or casein protein, fat-free or dry milk)

11% sugars (any blend of sucrose, high-fructose corn syrup, fructose, and corn-syrup solids)

80.5% water

The "milk drink" is the dairy industry equivalent of the "juice cocktail." You think you're paying for a protein-dense dose of moo juice, perhaps spiked with a bit of chocolate to make it go down easier, but instead you're looking at a bottle or carton dominated by plain old water. Worse than that, in an attempt to simulate a milk-like texture, you end up with a mess of thickeners and stabilizers and even a bit of trans fat in the form of partially hydrogenated oil.

SOFT DRINKS
Drink This

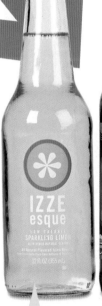

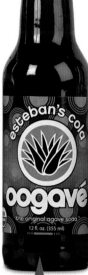

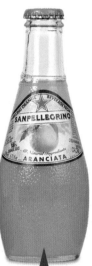

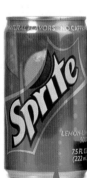

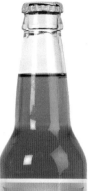

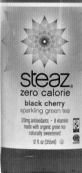

Izze Esque Sparkling Limon
(12 fl oz)

50 calories
0 g fat
11 g sugars

Our favorite drink on this page, made from 25% juice, sparkling water, and natural flavoring.

Oogavé Esteban's Cola
(12 fl oz)

102 calories
0 g fat
24 g sugars

Truth is, you'd be better off going diet, but if you're going to indulge, you may as well let Esteban give you your fix and save 38 calories.

San Pellegrino Aranciata
(6.75 fl oz)

80 calories
0 g fat
19 g sugars

Any drink with real juice trumps a soda every time. This one has 18% of the real stuff, plus a perfect portion size to boot.

Sprite
(7.5 fl oz)

90 calories
0 g fat
24 g sugars

Thanks to soda manufacturers for finally going back to the smaller serving sizes of yesteryear. It's still a bad drink, you just have less of it doing damage.

Steaz Zero Calorie Black Cherry Sparkling Green Tea
(12 fl oz)

0 calories
0 g fat
0 g sugars

Harnesses tea's nutritional powers without the sugars.

Let's get one thing straight: Very few of these drinks have any redeeming nutritional value at all. You'd be best to cut soft drinks out of your life entirely, but if you find yourself with a craving for carbonation, the drinks on the left side will do the least amount of damage.

Not That!

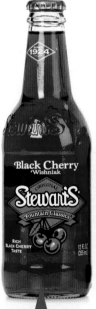

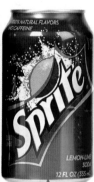

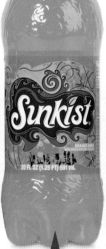

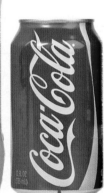

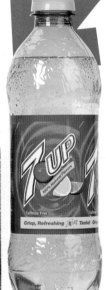

Stewart's Black Cherry
(12 fl oz)

190 calories
0 g fat
46 g sugars

Don't be fooled by fancy throwback bottles. More often than not, the liquid inside is more sugar-laden than normal sodas.

Sprite
(12 fl oz)

140 calories
0 g fat
38 g sugars

Do you really need those extra 4.5 ounces? For that matter, do you really need a Sprite at all with so many tasty, healthy alternatives out there?

Sunkist
(per 8 fl oz)

130 calories
0 g fat
34 g sugars

Ounce for ounce, the worst soft drink on the market today.

Coca-Cola
(12 fl oz)

140 calories
0 g fat
39 g sugars

Our US companies sure can export obesity. Coke is consumed in more than 200 countries.

7Up
(per 12 fl oz)

150 calories
0 g fat
38 g sugars

Izze provides the same satisfying lemon-lime combination, but does so with real juice, not high-fructose corn syrup and "natural flavoring."

121

Chapter

4

Drink This, Not That!

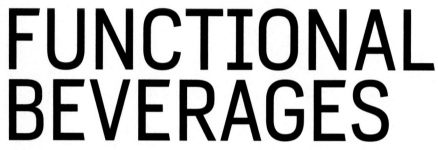

FUNCTIONAL BEVERAGES

Home-run hitters!
Viruses!
Governors of California!
Octomoms!
Features on Heidi Montag's face!

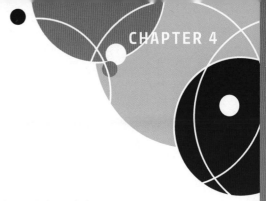

CHAPTER 4

Slow down, evolution! Is there anything left on Earth that hasn't suddenly become a turbo-boosted, supercharged, over-the-top, performance-driven facsimile of what it once was? Is there anyone who remembers a time when baseball players had nicknames like "The Splendid Splinter," politicians didn't need tailoring to help their shirts fit over their biceps, and mom was more likely to have a dozen cupcakes in the oven than a dozen embryos in the freezer?

Of course, there's something uniquely American about our quest to want to constantly get better, progress forward, reinvent ourselves. Heck, it took us only 200 years to go from having an American president who owned Africans to having an African-American who became president. (By contrast, it took the French that long just to build the Chartres Cathedral. And they didn't even have to do an end-run around the Clintons to get there!)

Perhaps it was inevitable then that all this constant tweaking and improving and reinventing of ourselves and our culture would eventually affect even the foods and beverages we consume. Now, thanks to our continually turbo-charging state of mind, the shelves of our supermarkets, gyms, and bodegas are filled with "high-performance" or "functional" beverages. But what function, exactly, are these beverages performing?

Some will help you build muscle. Some will help you stay awake and alert. And many of them—too many of them—will help you grow fat. Consider, if you will, the case of the "energy drink."

The original energy drink—a cup of black coffee—comes with a payload of energizing caffeine and a mere 2 calories. But let's say regular joe isn't good enough for you—you want to turbocharge your energy boost, and pick up one of those chemical-experiments-in-a-can. A 16-ounce can of Rockstar Original will cost you 280 calories—140 times as much as coffee!—and load you up with 62 grams of teeth-rattling, insulin-insulting refined sugar. Swapping just one Rockstar for one cup of coffee each day means enough additional calories to add nearly 29 pounds to your body a year.

What if a real rock star like, say, Keith Richards, did that? Let's see, the Rolling Stones started in 1962, so one Rockstar Original a day since then would mean that Richards would now weigh . . . 1,391 pounds more!

See, not every "functional" beverage functions quite the way we want it to. And that holds true whether the "function" is to give you energy, help you recuperate from a workout, protect your immune system, or just turn you into a giant sloshing vat of liquid vitamins. Before you buy the hype—before you start thinking that drinking Rockstar or Monster or Shark will turn you into one—read the following.

The Truth About Functional Beverages

In the 19th century, traveling "doctors" would float from town to town peddling new-fangled elixirs. They'd gather crowds and promise miracle cures for everything from wrinkled skin to chronic disease. And if the crowd seemed unconvinced, some pawn in the audience would stand up and testify to the potency of the charlatan's potion.

Today we refer to these men as snake-oil salesmen, and their techniques seem to have been appropriated for the budding functional beverage market. Think about it: The ads feature both doctors and paid testimonies—the salesman and the pawn—and the bottles feature overblown health claims—the miracle cure. Between the elaborate vitamin packages and exotic-sounding extracts, it's hard to tell if you're drinking sugar water or a tonic for life everlasting. Read on to see how to separate a sincere health claim from a snake-oil sales pitch.

Jones GABA Lemon Honey

THE CLAIM

"Focus + Clarity"

"GABA (or gamma-aminobutyric acid, for you scientific types) enhances mental focus, balance, and clarity. It helps increase production of calming alpha brain waves and decrease beta brain waves, which are linked to nervousness and scattered thoughts."

THE TRUTH

There's no question about whether GABA will make you feel calm. It is, after all, among the most abundant neurotransmitters at work in your brain, and its effect can be thought of as the opposite of caffeine—soothing, tranquilizing, and relaxing. The thing is, your body produces the stuff naturally, and nobody has been able to prove that the GABA you take orally will ever reach your brain. That's not to say the chemical doesn't have its advocates. Many bodybuilders swear by the stuff, but that's because it's thought to increase the body's production of growth hormones and aid in muscle recovery. But the evidence for this, too, is more anecdotal than scientific.

IS IT SAFE?

There's no reason to doubt the safety of GABA, but as to whether it will produce the desired results, the jury's still out. And while the smaller can size ensures a lighter dose of sugar, we can't advocate giving up 90 calories for a drink that may or may not have any benefit for you.

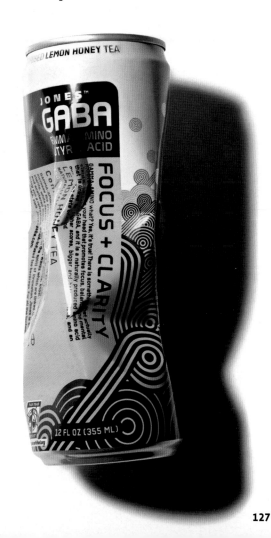

Snapple Antioxidant Water Awaken Dragonfruit

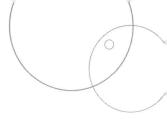

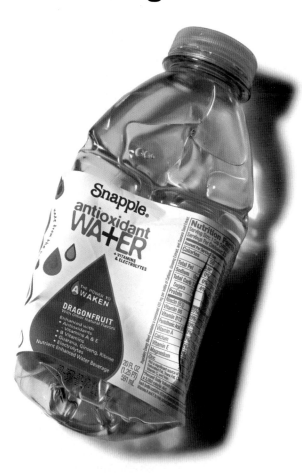

THE CLAIM

"A fireworks display of natural stimulants like guarana, ginseng, and caffeine to awaken your body with a chorus of oooohs and aaaahs."

THE TRUTH

Whereas some functional beverages take the rifle approach—one vitamin or herb loaded in the barrel to target one area of your well-being—Snapple's bottle follows a shotgun strategy: a hodgepodge of nutrients and extracts stuffed in with the hope that something will achieve the desired result. This is the same technique favored by most energy-drink companies. Guarana, ginseng, and caffeine are the same triad used by brands like Rockstar and Monster, and Snapple also relies on a heft of B vitamins to work its energy-inducing magic. What this bottle has that the energy drinks don't is a green-tea compound called EGCG, epigallo-catechin gallate, which is a well-established, disease-fighting antioxidant. That being said, there's still a touch of the old snake-oil to this bottle. Vitamins A and E, touted on the front label, won't do much good considering they're fat-soluble and this bottle contains not a lick of fat.

IS IT SAFE?

Aside from the 125 calories of sugar in each bottle, yes it's safe. The only groups who might use caution are those taking other medications. The ginseng might disrupt the function of the blood-thinning drug warfarin.

Glacéau Vitaminwater Defense Raspberry-Apple

THE CLAIM

"Vitamins + Water = All you need"

"Specially formulated with nutrients required for optimal functioning of the immune system."

THE TRUTH

The keystone of all Vitaminwater products is a barrage of B vitamins, but any boon this bottle provides to your immune system is coming from two primary ingredients: vitamin C and zinc. The first, vitamin C, has a reputation for fighting the common cold, but studies don't fully support the claim. Researchers in Finland examined 30 of these studies and found that vitamin C supplements benefited only one small group of people: those under extreme physical stress. The rest of us do fine with the surplus of vitamin C we get from everyday foods. Zinc, on the other hand, might be a little more promising. A recent study at the University of Florida found that daily zinc supplementation could increase the body's production of T cells, which help the body fight viral and bacterial infections. Problem is, the study used a daily dose of 15 milligrams—about four times as much as you get from a bottle of Defense.

IS IT SAFE?

As safe as a multivitamin and 6 spoonfuls of sugar. Whatever benefit you receive won't outweigh the 125-calorie investment. If you truly are sick, then the water in this bottle will probably do more good than the vitamins.

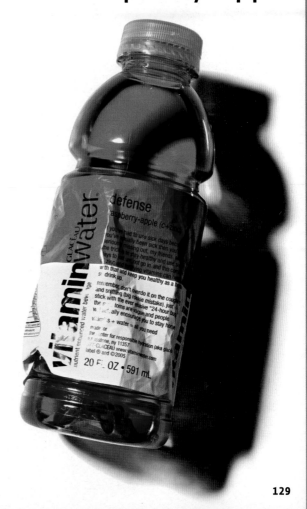

Function: Urban Detox

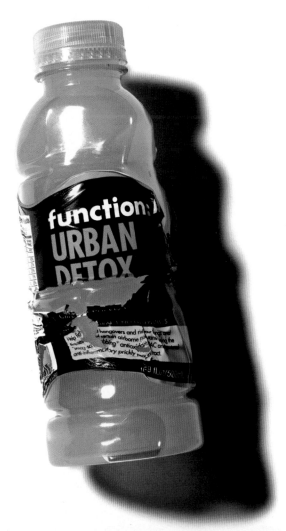

"Urban Detox is designed to support healthy lungs and sinuses in the face of particulate airborne pollution. These same ingredients support the liver's efforts in combating hangovers."

THE TRUTH

If this is your only defense against city smog, then consider yourself underprotected, but when it comes to hangover remedies, this bottle might actually deliver. Researchers in New Orleans found that subjects given prickly pear extract, one of the compounds at work in this bottle, experienced fewer hangover symptoms after a night of heavy drinking. The subjects took the supplement before drinking, and the next morning they were less nauseous, had fewer instances of dry mouth, and had stronger appetites than their placebo-taking peers. Forget to guzzle a bottle before hitting the booze? That's okay, too. Among the dose of B vitamins found in this bottle is four times your daily value of B_6, a vitamin that tends to suffer depletion at the hands of a long night of drinking. It might not be a perfect cure, but this—along with a greasy omelet—is as good a shot as you've got.

IS IT SAFE?

Sure it carries a potent dose of B vitamins, but it's not nearly enough to induce toxicity symptoms. The bigger question is whether this vitamin cocktail is worth the 100-calorie cost. Maybe in emergency situations (read: after a serious bender), but your best antidote remains a whole lot of H_2O.

SoBe Lifewater Strawberry Kiwi Bliss

THE CLAIM

"Stressed? Feel groovy
with our soothing strawberry
and kiwi-flavored drink,
with lemon balm and hibiscus."

THE TRUTH

Happiness in a bottle? That's a tough pill to swallow. Especially when you consider how SoBe plans to make it happen. Aside from the standard B vitamins that lace nearly every functional beverage on the market, this one has the added bonus of two extracts: lemon balm and hibiscus. The good new is, one of these herbs has a high likelihood of reducing stress. The bad news? There's probably not enough of it in this bottle for you to notice. In a British study, subjects who received 600-milligram doses of lemon balm every day for a week reported feeling significantly more calm at the study's end. The tradeoff was they also felt less alert. So how much lemon balm is in this beverage? SoBe isn't saying, but you can bet your bottle it's less than 600 milligrams. As for hibiscus, its only real value is in its ability to fight hypertension. Clinical studies have shown it to lower blood pressure, but generally it's tested in concentrations at or near 10 grams per day. Again, that's far more than you can expect to find in this bottle.

IS IT SAFE?

The low levels of vitamins and presumably low levels of extracts make this as harmless as sweet herbal tea. It has slightly less sugar than some of the other bottles on the shelf, but water and sugar are still the first two ingredients, which make it more treat than treatment.

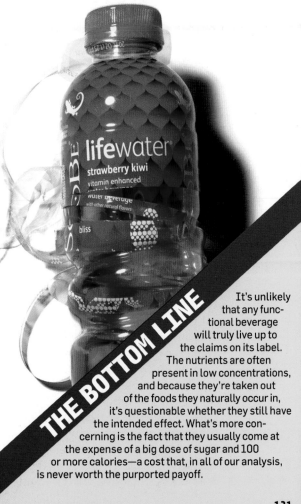

THE BOTTOM LINE

It's unlikely that any functional beverage will truly live up to the claims on its label. The nutrients are often present in low concentrations, and because they're taken out of the foods they naturally occur in, it's questionable whether they still have the intended effect. What's more concerning is the fact that they usually come at the expense of a big dose of sugar and 100 or more calories—a cost that, in all of our analysis, is never worth the purported payoff.

Energy or Enemy?

Analyzing the health implications of this country's ever-growing energy-drink obsession

Energy drinks sell you on increasing alertness, fighting fatigue, and improving reaction time. But we wondered: When you pop the top, what are you really pouring into your body?

Apparently, it doesn't take a biochemist to formulate an energy drink. No, according to Starbucks, any guy off the street is qualified. At least, that's whose opinion mattered most when the coffee giant created the ingredient list for its own concoction.

"There are many energy ingredients on the market, and B vitamins, guarana, and ginseng are the ones our customers are most familiar with," says Ruby Amegah, product-development manager for the team behind the Starbucks Doubleshot Energy + Coffee.

Which perhaps in large part explains why the company chose them: It's smart marketing.

Trouble is, by letting consumer research influence ingredient lists, energy-drink companies are helping popularize exotic-sounding compounds that even scientists don't yet fully understand. The approach has worked: Last year, Americans spent $4.2 billion on these supposedly high-octane elixirs.

But do these beverages really energize your body and sharpen your mind? Or should you can the energy drinks for good? To help you separate the science from the marketing hype, we analyzed five key ingredients in the market's most popular potions.

Energy Ingredients

Ginseng

What Is It? An extract made from the root of the ginseng plant. Panax ginseng is the species most commonly used. The ginseng content in energy drinks typically ranges between 8 milligrams and 400 milligrams in 16 ounces.

Does It Work? Not if you're hoping for energy to burn. A recent review in *American Family Physician* determined that ginseng doesn't enhance physical performance. But there is an upside: It may boost your brainpower. Andrew Scholey, PhD, an herb and nutrition researcher at Australia's Swinburne University, and his colleagues found that people who swallowed 200 milligrams of the extract an hour before taking a cognitive test scored significantly better than when they skipped the supplement. They also felt less mental fatigue. Ginseng may work by increasing the uptake of blood glucose by cells in the brain, says Scholey. However, the right amount is essential—only two of the eight major energy drinks we examined contained that optimal dose of at least 200 milligrams.

Is It Safe? Because the amount of ginseng in an energy drink is minimal, harmful effects are unlikely. And while there have been some reports of negative side effects from ginseng—diarrhea, for example—Scholey points out that those occurred in people taking 3 grams a day. One caution: If you're on any medications, check with your doctor before knocking back an energy drink. Ginseng has been shown to impede blood-thinning drugs like warfarin.

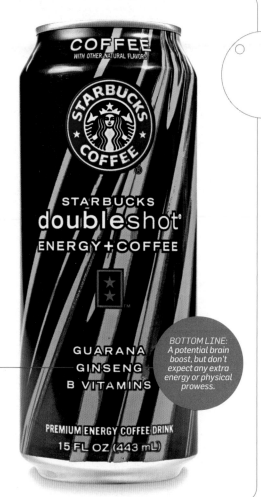

BOTTOM LINE: A potential brain boost, but don't expect any extra energy or physical prowess.

Energy Ingredients

Guarana

What Is It? A South American shrub. One seed has a caffeine content of 4 to 5 percent, while a coffee bean has 1 to 2 percent. The amount of guarana in a 16-ounce energy drink ranges from a minuscule 1.4 milligrams to as much as 300 milligrams.

Does It Work? Yes, if you don't set the bar too high. A study in the journal *Appetite* reports that people who took 222 milligrams of guarana felt slightly less fatigued and were up to 30 milliseconds faster on a reaction-time test than those who popped a placebo. Some scientists attribute guarana's effect solely to its caffeine content, but Scholey isn't so sure. His team found energizing effects with doses just under 40 milligrams, which contains little caffeine. That means there's probably something else in guarana that produces a stimulating effect on its own or that bolsters the effect of the caffeine, he says.

Is It Safe? Scientists at Florida's Nova Southeastern University recently conducted tests and concluded that the amounts of guarana found in most energy drinks aren't large enough to cause any adverse effects. That said, there's still a question mark regarding the safety of higher levels, which could conceivably be consumed by downing a few energy drinks in a brief time span.

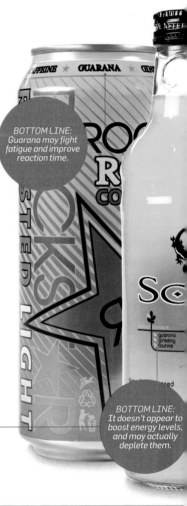

BOTTOM LINE: Guarana may fight fatigue and improve reaction time.

Taurine

What Is It? One of the most abundant amino acids in your brain, where it can act as a neurotransmitter—a chemical messenger that allows your cells to communicate with one another. You'll find anywhere from 20 milligrams to 2,000 milligrams of taurine in most 16-ounce energy drinks.

Does It Work? Scientists aren't sure, but it doesn't seem likely. When taurine is dumped into your bloodstream—when you down a Red Bull, for instance—it can't pass through the membranes that protect your brain, says Neil Harrison, PhD, a professor of pharmacology at Weill Cornell Medical College. But even if it could, Harrison's research suggests that taurine might behave more like a sedative than a stimulant. When he and his team applied the amino acid to the brain tissue of rodents, they discovered that it mimicked a neurotransmitter that slows brain activity.

Is It Safe? Taurine is probably fine in small doses, but chug too many energy drinks and the picture becomes less clear. According to a recent case report from St. Joseph's Hospital in Phoenix, Arizona, three people had seizures after drinking two 24-ounce energy drinks in a short period of time. However, the researchers don't know whether to blame the taurine or the caffeine. The fact is, there's been little research on taurine consumption in humans, so it's impossible to conclude whether it's safe to consume in high doses.

BOTTOM LINE: It doesn't appear to boost energy levels, and may actually deplete them.

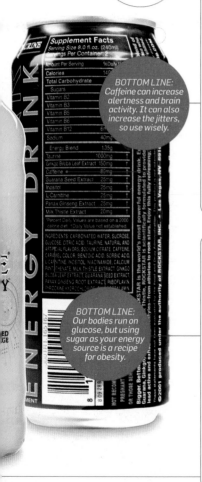

Supplement Facts
Serving Size 8.0 fl.oz. (240ml)
Servings Per Container: 2

Amount Per Serving	%Daily V...
Calories	140
Total Carbohydrate	
Sugars	
Vitamin B2	
Vitamin B3	
Vitamin B5	
Vitamin B6	
Vitamin B12	6...
Sodium	40mg
Energy Blend	135g
Taurine	1000mg
Ginkgo Biloba Leaf Extract	150mg †
Caffeine	80mg †
Guarana Seed Extract	25mg †
Inositol	25mg †
L-Carnitine	25mg †
Panax Ginseng Extract	25mg †
Milk Thistle Extract	20mg †

*Percent Daily Values are based on a 2000 calorie diet. †Daily Value not established.

INGREDIENTS: CARBONATED WATER, SUCROSE, GLUCOSE, CITRIC ACID, TAURINE, NATURAL AND ARTIFICIAL FLAVORS, SODIUM CITRATE, CAFFEINE, CARAMEL COLOR, BENZOIC ACID, SORBIC ACID, L-CARNITINE, INOSITOL, NIACINAMIDE, CALCIUM PANTOTHENATE, MILK THISTLE EXTRACT, GINKGO BILOBA LEAF EXTRACT, GUARANA SEED EXTRACT, PANAX GINSENG ROOT EXTRACT, RIBOFLAVIN, PYRIDOXINE HYDROCHLORIDE...

BOTTOM LINE: *Caffeine can increase alertness and brain activity. It can also increase the jitters, so use wisely.*

BOTTOM LINE: *Our bodies run on glucose, but using sugar as your energy source is a recipe for obesity.*

Caffeine

What Is It? A chemical compound that stimulates your central nervous system. Most energy drinks contain between 140 and 170 milligrams of caffeine in a 15- or 16-ounce can.

Does It Work? Java junkies certainly think so. As for the science, an Austrian study showed that men who swallowed 100 milligrams of caffeine had a bigger boost in brain activity after 20 minutes than those who took a placebo. Plus, a new University of Chicago study found that a 200-milligram jolt made fatigued people feel twice as alert as noncaffeinated participants.

Is It Safe? The most caffeine-packed energy drink contains the equivalent in caffeine of about two 8-ounce cups of coffee. If downing that much joe doesn't make you jittery, then quaffing a can shouldn't pose a problem. Of course, if you combine that with other caffeinated beverages throughout the day, then the sum total stimulation could cause headaches, sleeplessness, or nausea. On the other hand, if you're not a regular coffee or cola drinker and you battle high blood pressure, the occasional energy drink could be trouble. Researchers in Finland reported that the caffeine in 2 to 3 cups of coffee can cause blood pressure to spike by up to 14 points.

Glucose

What Is It? Sugar. Sucrose, another ingredient you'll often see on energy drink labels, is a combination of fructose (the natural sugar found in fruit) and glucose. Many energy drinks contain 50 to 60 grams of glucose or sucrose in a 16-ounce can.

Does It Work? Your body runs mainly on glucose, so topping off your tank with the sweet stuff should theoretically provide an instant boost. And in fact, a recent study in the *Journal of Applied Physiology* found that men who guzzled a 6 percent glucose drink were able to bicycle 22 minutes longer than those who went sans the extra sugar. Where glucose won't help, however, is with the fog of fatigue from too little sleep. A 2006 British study determined that sleep-deprived people who drank liquid glucose exhibited slower reaction times and more sleepiness after 90 minutes than those who drank nothing.

Is It Safe? Dumping empty calories down your gullet is never a great idea, and some energy drinks contain nearly as much sugar as a 20-ounce soda. Then there's the fact that a sudden infusion of glucose can cause your blood sugar and insulin levels to skyrocket, signaling your body to stop incinerating fat. A 2006 New Zealand study reveals that caffeine combined with even the 27 grams of sugar in, say, an 8.3-ounce Red Bull may be enough to temporarily inhibit your body's ability to burn lard.

Drink This

The fastest-expanding niche in the beverage industry is also among the most problematic.

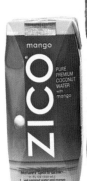

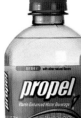

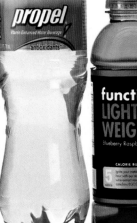

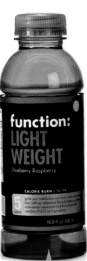

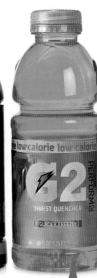

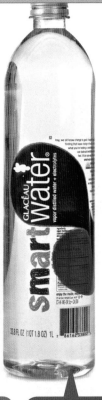

Zico Pure Coconut Water Mango
(11 fl oz container)

60 calories
0 g fat
14 g sugars

Coconut water offers the electrolytes of Gatorade with less sugar and no artificial add-ins.

Propel Berry
(24 fl oz bottle)

30 calories
0 g fat
6 g sugars

The original functional beverage is also among the best. It's low in sugar, contains no artificial coloring, and carries a bevy of vitamins.

Function: Light Weight Blueberry Raspberry
(16.9 fl oz bottle)

11 calories
0 g fat
2 g sugars

This bottle boasts both EGCG and resveratrol, the star nutrients from the world of tea and wine.

Gatorade G2 Glacier Freeze
(20 fl oz bottle)

45 calories
0 g fat
12 g sugars

Fewer than half the calories of traditional Gatorade, but with all the same electrolytes to encourage full hydration.

Glacéau Smart Water
(33.8 fl oz bottle)

0 calories
0 g fat
0 g sugars

Zero sugar, zero calories. Just water and electrolytes. Now that's refreshing.

Not That!

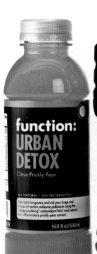

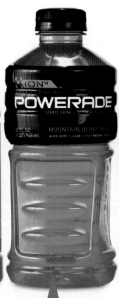

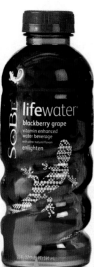

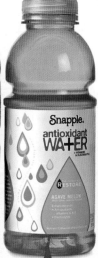

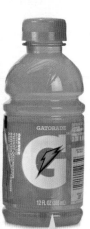

Function: Urban Detox Citrus Prickly Pear
(16.9 fl oz bottle)

100 calories
0 g fat
24 g sugars

It may help with a hangover, but so does water, and that won't cost you more than a few pennies.

Powerade Mountain Berry Blast
(32 fl oz bottle)

200 calories
0 g fat
56 g sugars

You'd need to run 2 miles to work this off. Save 200 calories by switching to sucralose-sweetened Powerade Zero.

SoBe Lifewater Blackberry Grape Enlighten
(20 fl oz bottle)

90 calories
0 g fat
23 g sugars

Any "water" with more than 20 grams of sugar has no place in your diet.

Snapple Antioxidant Water Agave Melon
(20 fl oz bottle)

140 calories
0 g fat
32 g sugars

This "water," packs as many calories as a can of 7Up. We like our antioxidants sans sucrose.

Gatorade G Orange
(12 fl oz bottle)

80 calories
0 g fat
21 g sugars

Loads of artificial coloring and high-fructose corn syrup compromise an otherwise admirable beverage.

Drink This

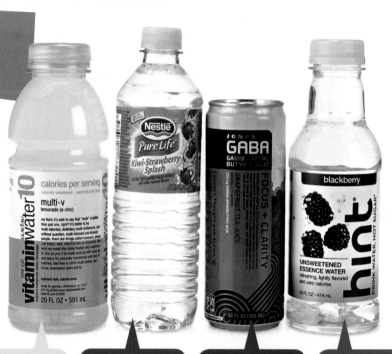

Glacéau Vitamin Water 10 Lemonade Multi-V
(20 fl oz bottle)

25 calories
0 g fat
7.5 g sugars

The new 10 line replaces sugar with rebiana, a noncaloric sweetener from the stevia plant.

Nestlé Pure Life Kiwi-Strawberry Splash
(16 fl oz bottle)

0 calories
0 g fat
0 g sugars

Carries a splash of natural flavoring and sucralose to help you break your sugar-loaded drinking habits.

Jones GABA Focus + Clarity Grapefruit
(12 fl oz can)

80 calories
0 g fat
19 g sugars

Not a light beverage by any means, but the 12-ounce can tampers the sugar's potential to cause serious damage.

Hint Blackberry
(16 fl oz bottle)

0 calories
0 g fat
0 g sugars

Hint is one of the best finds out there for people who want a bit of flavor with their water. Its slogan: Drink water, not sugar. We couldn't agree more.

Not That!

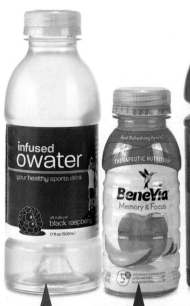

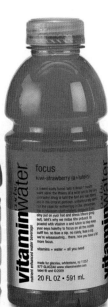

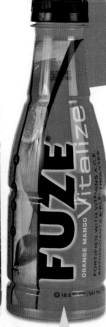

Infused Owater Black Raspberry
(17 fl oz bottle)
72 calories
0 g fat
19 g sugars

This falls in the middle of the pack when it comes to "enhanced" waters. But when it comes to water, 72 calories is still about 72 too many.

BeneVia Memory and Focus
(8 fl oz container)
160 calories
0 g fat
31 g sugars

This is the most calorie-dense functional beverage we've seen. It's hard to imagine someone being able to focus with so much sugar coursing through his or her veins.

Glacéau Vitamin Water Focus Kiwi-Strawberry
(20 fl oz bottle)
125 calories
0 g fat
32.5 g sugars

Adding just one of these to your daily intake will put 13 pounds on your body in a year.

Fuze Vitalize Orange Mango
(18.5 fl oz bottle)
209 calories
0 g fat
58 g sugars

It carries stout loads of vitamins A and E, but it's not nearly worth the caloric damage.

139

ENERGY DRINKS

Drink This

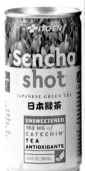

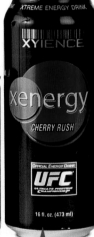

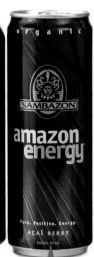

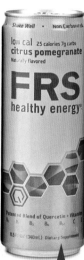

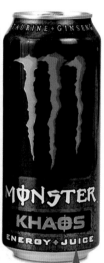

Ito En Sencha Shot
(6.4 fl oz can)

0 calories
0 g fat
0 sugars

The green-tea-based catechins in this bottle have been linked to weight loss and heart-disease prevention.

Xenergy Cherry Rush
(16 fl oz can)

0 calories
0 g fat
0 sugars

If it's prolonged energy you seek, sugar will only slow you down. Xenergy delivers the punch of guarana without any of the sweet stuff.

Sambazon Energy Açai Berry
(12 fl oz can)

120 calories
0 g fat
28.5 g sugars

Carries a dose of caffeine plus antioxidant-rich açai juice and the extracts of yerba mate and green tea.

FRS Healthy Energy Low Cal Citrus Pomegranate
(11.5 fl oz can)

25 calories
0 g fat
4 g sugars

Sweetened with real juice and packing a couple grams of fiber. It's tough to find a better energy drink.

Monster Khaos
(16 fl oz can)

140 calories
0 g fat
34 g sugars

With half its calories coming from fruit juice, Khaos has nutritional heft that goes beyond just B vitamins.

Not That!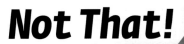

*Just remember:
Cans heavy in sugar will ultimately
only serve to slow you down.*

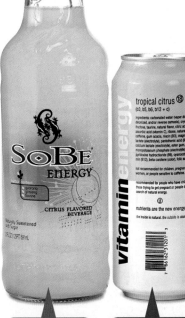

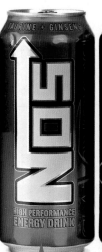

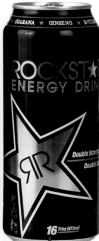

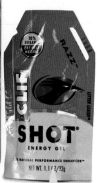

SoBe Energy Citrus Flavored Beverage
(20 fl oz bottle)

270 calories
0 g fat
66 g sugars

Has more sugar than three scoops of Baskin-Robbins Cookies 'n' Cream Ice Cream.

Glaceau Vitamin Energy Tropical Citrus
(16 fl oz can)

200 calories
0 g fat
50 g sugars

Even more sugar-laden than Glaceau's disappointing Vitamin Water drinks.

NOS Energy
(16 fl oz can)

220 calories
0 g fat
52 g sugars

No amount of energy is worth more than 200 calories. Go with a lighter beverage or a smaller can.

Rockstar
(16 fl oz can)

280 calories
0 g fat
62 g sugars

The most sugar-concentrated of all the energy drinks.

Clif Razz Energy Gel Shot
(32 g package)

100 calories
0 g fat
8 g sugars

Beware the gel-based "energy" shots. Most of their potential is actually wrapped up in fast-burning carbs.

Drink This

Whether it's weight loss, appetite control, or muscle growth you seek, look for shakes high in protein and fiber and low in sugar.

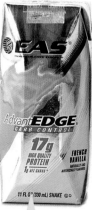
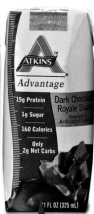
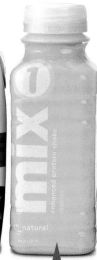
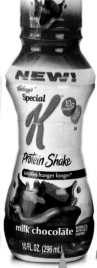
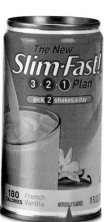

EAS AdvantEdge Carb Control French Vanilla
(11 fl oz container)

110 calories
3 g fat
(0 g saturated)
0 g sugars

Delivers 17 grams of protein and a heft of essential minerals.

Atkins Advantage Dark Chocolate Royale
(11 fl oz bottle)

160 calories
9 g fat
(1.5 g saturated)
1 g sugars

Attacks hunger, not your blood sugar.

Mix 1 All-Natural Protein Mango
(11 fl oz bottle)

200 calories
2.5 g fat
(0 g saturated)
22 g sugars

Packs 15 grams of whey protein, plus a dose of metabolism-boosting green tea polyphenols.

Special K Protein Shake Milk Chocolate
(10 fl oz bottle)

190 calories
5 g fat
(0.5 g saturated)
18 g sugars

This is surprisingly good—especially considering the low quality of many of Special K's cereals.

Slim-Fast! French Vanilla
(11 fl oz can)

180 calories
6 g fat
(1.5 g saturated)
18 g sugars

The classic weight-loss shake curbs hunger with a respectable 10 grams of protein and 5 grams of fiber.

Not That!

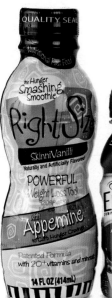

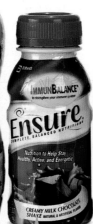

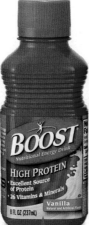

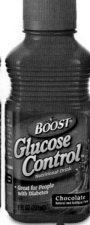

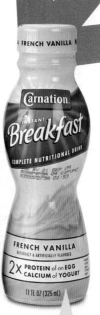

Right Size SkinniVanilli
(14 fl oz bottle)

263 calories
5.5 g fat
(2.5 g saturated)
30 g sugars

The Skinni sell is hard to swallow when it comes with as much sugar as two scoops of Breyers vanilla ice cream.

Ensure Creamy Milk Chocolate Shake
(8 fl oz bottle)

250 calories
6 g fat
(1 g saturated)
22 g sugars

The second ingredient is sugar followed by corn-based carbs.

Boost High Protein Vanilla
(8 fl oz bottle)

240 calories
6 g fat
(0.5 g saturated)
18 g sugars

The same amount of protein as Mix 1's version, but with 40 more calories from sugar and fat.

Boost Glucose Control Chocolate
(8 fl oz bottle)

190 calories
7 g fat
(1 g saturated)
4 g sugars

If you're trying to keep your blood sugar in check, Atkins does the job better with less sugar and more fiber.

Carnation Instant Breakfast Essentials French Vanilla
(11 fl oz bottle)

250 calories
5 g fat
(1.5 g saturated)
31 g sugars

As much sugar as four Peanut Butter Twix bars.

143

Drink This

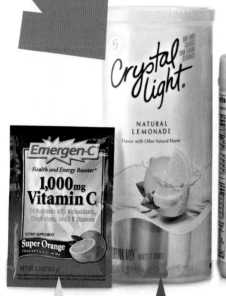
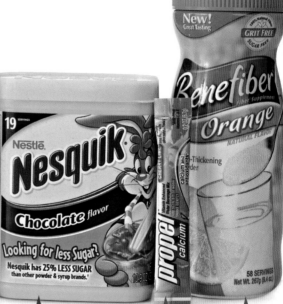

Emergen-C Super Orange
(8 fl oz prepared)

25 calories
0 g fat
5 g sugars

You get Gatorade's electrolytes for a fraction of the caloric cost, plus more than 1,000% of your daily vitamin C.

Crystal Light Natural Lemon
(8 fl oz prepared)

5 calories
0 g fat
0 g sugars

Crystal Light is one of the most reliable low-calorie powders around. Find it in just about any supermarket.

Nesquik Chocolate
(8 fl oz prepared)

60 calories
0.5 g fat
(0 g saturated)
13 g sugars

Nesquik also makes a great sugar-free powder, which knocks 25 calories off the caloric price tag.

Propel Cherry Lime
(16.9 fl oz prepared)

20 calories
0 g fat
4 g sugars

Propel trounces Kool-Aid with a two-pronged approach: It cuts the sugar and eliminates the artificial coloring.

Benefiber Orange
(4 to 8 fl oz prepared)

15 calories
0 g fat
0 g sugars

This is a great new product from Benefiber. It provides a nice orange flavor with 3 grams of heart-healthy fiber.

Not That!

Powdered beverages are a good way to stretch a buck. But if you're not careful in establishing your allegiances, they're also a good way to stretch a waistline.

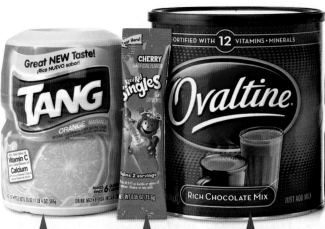

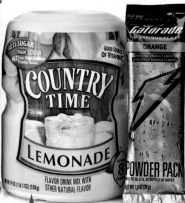

Tang Orange
(8 fl oz prepared)

90 calories
0 g fat
22 g sugars

Here's a dependable rule to help you lose weight: Don't drink anything that provides nary a shred of nutritional value.

Kool-Aid Cherry
(8 fl oz prepared)

60 calories
0 g fat
16 g sugars

Don't expect much from a brand that built its reputation around an obese glass jug that broke through walls.

Ovaltine Rich Chocolate
(8 fl oz prepared)

80 calories
0 g fat
18 g sugars

Ovaltine's chocolate granules are weaker than Nesquik's, which is why it takes twice as much to achieve the same flavor.

Country Time Lemonade
(8 fl oz prepared)

60 calories
0 g fat
16 g sugars

First ingredient is sugar. Second ingredient? Fructose—aka more sugar.

Gatorade Orange
(8 fl oz prepared)

50 calories
0 g fat
14 g sugars

The only source of energy in Gatorade is sugar. Find a better sports drink.

145

5

Drink This, Not That!

JUICE & SMOOTHIES

Question:
What does Lindsay Lohan
have in common with
a glass of orange juice?

CHAPTER 5

Answer:

Both are sort of orange-colored.

Okay, yes, that's true, but we were actually looking for something more substantial here. Let's try again.

Answer number two: Both orange juice and Lindsay Lohan were once considered sweet, wholesome, and good for you. But like the flame-haired former Disney star, orange juice too has been revealed to have a dark side—and spending too much time with either can be bad for your health.

That sounds a bit counterintuitive. After all, fruit is good for you. Juice comes from fruit. So, juice must be good for you, too. But juice without the fruit it came from is like David Lee Roth without the band he came from: The tangy flavor is still there, but a lot of the substance is missing. And in the case of juice, the substance that's missing is, primarily, hunger-quenching fiber. For example, a study published in the *American Journal of Clinical Nutrition* looked at how satisfying a 65-calorie orange was compared to a 6-ounce glass of orange juice (which clocked in at 85 calories). Sixty minutes after their snack, those who drank juice were starting to get hungry, yet those who ate the fruit weren't. An hour after that, the juice drinkers were really feeling empty, while the orange eaters were still totally satisfied. (Exactly comparable to the feeling you get after hearing "Just a Gigolo" versus "Running with the Devil." Amazing!) The reason is simple: When you juice a fruit, what's strained out is all the belly-filling fiber. And the real bummer is that you not only miss the hunger-quenching benefits of that fiber, but you also don't get to enjoy the fruit as much either: One study found that people consume juice 11 times faster than whole fruit. Talk about a moment on the lips!

But not all fruit drinks are nutritional downers. By mixing calcium-rich yogurt and vitamin- and fiber-packed fruit, a good smoothie can deliver nutrients the way Drew Brees delivers touchdown passes—right into your hands. (Plus, there's nothing more satisfying than the Jimmy Buffet vibe you get from tossing stuff into a blender and hitting "puree.") And a good smoothie keeps you satisfied: In one study, European researchers gave participants either a low-calorie fruit drink, a high-carb fruit drink, or a smoothie with whey protein. Then they sent all three groups to the buffet table. The result: The subjects who drank the smoothies ate less than the other two groups—about 80 fewer calories. But pick carefully: Many of the smoothies in these pages are junk food in disguise. By knowing which smoothies and fruit drinks to pick, you'll start stripping away flab and boosting your overall health—all while drinking down dessert.

If only Lindsay Lohan's troubles could be so easily solved…

The Ultimate Smoothie Selector

Unless you've been living in an igloo for the past two decades, you should know by now that Americans do not eat enough fruits and vegetables. In fact, recent surveys have found that only about 30 percent of Americans are eating the recommended 5 or more servings of fruits and vegetables a day. That's a pretty pitiful performance and no doubt a partial cause of the obesity epidemic that grips this nation.

If you happen to be one of those 7 out of 10 of us who don't eat enough plant matter, then you need to make fast friends with the smoothie. It's the quickest, most delicious way to make up for the fruit-and-vegetable deficit: Roll out of bed, toss some fruit in a blender, top with a bit of liquid, hit "liquefy." Boom! You're on

Over the years, the line between smoothie and milk shake has been irrevocably blurred by the beverage industry. What was once a reliable, all-fruit concoction is now likely to be an ice-cream-and-added-sugar extravaganza, capable of carrying over 2,000 calories a serving (see Smoothie King, Hulk). For about a buck a glass, you can take all of the guesswork out of the smoothie conundrum and ensure yourself instant access to a bona fide healthy beverage. Consider these your blueprints.

the path to a skinnier, healthier existence.

Making smoothies can be a pretty free-wheeling endeavor, which is certainly part of the fun, but we've established a few basic rules. Follow these and the ingredient-by-ingredient guide that follows and you'll be ready for liquid liftoff.

Rule #1: No ice cream.
If you want ice cream in your smoothie, call it what it is—a milk shake—and have it for dessert.

Rule #2: Use a strong blender.
A weak blender won't be able to crush the ice quickly enough, which means it melts and ultimately dilutes your precious creation, rather than giving it that bracing, velvety texture you want.

Rule #3: Respect the ratio.
Once you learn the basic proportions of liquids to solids, you can turn anything into a pretty drinkable smoothie. For every 3 cups of fruit, you'll need about 1 cup of liquid. Keep in mind that both yogurt and ice will thicken your drink.

Rule #4: Look to the freezer.
Not only is frozen fruit considerably more affordable, but research has found that frozen fruits may actually carry higher levels of antioxidants because they're picked at the height of season and flash frozen on the spot. Also, frozen fruit means you can use less ice to make your smoothie sufficiently cold, which in turn yields a more intense, pure flavor.

Fruit

Mango

107 calories
24 g sugars
3 g fiber

This tropical treasure has become increasingly available in American supermarkets, in both fresh and frozen forms. Yes, it's higher in sugar than almost any other fruit in the produce section, but it also brings to the blender three-quarters of your day's vitamin C and 25 percent of your vitamin A. Consider added sweeteners entirely superfluous when making smoothies with mango.

Papaya

55 calories
8 g sugars
3 g fiber

Is there any fruit better for you than papaya? Flooded with vitamin C, replete with vision-strengthening vitamin A, and blessed with one of the most favorable fiber-to-sugar ratios imaginable, papaya proves itself to be one of the most well-rounded foods on the planet. Papaya also boasts papain and chymopapain, two potent enzymes that have been shown to fight inflammation, the cause of asthma, arthritis, and other serious conditions.

Blueberries

84 calories
15 g sugars
4 g fiber

Blueberries are best known in health circles for anthocyanins, the phytonutrients that give them their blue-red tint and their dense antioxidant punch. That punch translates into serious brain food, as blueberries have been found in studies to protect our noggins against both oxidative stress and the effects of age-related mental decay manifested in Alzheimer's and dementia.

Strawberries

49 calories
7 g sugars
3 g fiber

Beyond the monster dose of vitamin C (calorie for calorie, you'll get more C than you'd find in an orange), strawberries also prove to be a rich source of phenols, including the same brain-boosting, anti-inflammatory anthocyanins found in blueberries. They also lay claim to a rare and powerful antioxidant called ellagitannin, which has been shown to provide a stout defense against a variety of cancers.

Banana
(1 medium)

105 calories
14 g sugars
3 g fiber

Sure, there are fruits with deeper nutritional portfolios, but the humble banana serves as an all-star utility player in the smoothie game. Not only does it offer a handful of hard-to-find nutrients (heart-strengthening potassium, gut-friendly prebiotics), but it also provides smoothies with a balanced, creamy texture and enough natural sweetness to ensure no need for added sugar. Keep a few very ripe bananas in the freezer. When you're ready for a smoothie, slice off the peel and blend away.

Avocado
(1 medium Haas, peeled and pitted)

227 calories
21 g fat (3 g saturated)
9 g fiber

Avocado might not be a traditional smoothie constituent, but we're convinced that it should be. The calories come primarily from monounsaturated fat, the good stuff that protects your heart and helps beat back hunger. Add to that an impressive fiber load and you have the makings of a seriously satisfying smoothie.

Plus, avocados add a richness that makes it feel like you're splurging, even when you're not.

Pineapple

82 calories
16 g sugars
2 g fiber

Feeling low on energy? A cup of pineapple might just be the antidote. That's because pineapple is one of nature's best sources of manganese, a trace mineral that is essential for energy production. A cup provides 76 percent of your daily recommended intake, making pineapple nature's answer to Red Bull.

Peach

60 calories
13 g sugars
2 g fiber

Peaches pack lutein and zeaxanthin, powerful carotenoids proven to help protect your peepers from macular degeneration. Plus, the blast of beta carotene may help stave off heart disease and cancer. But a USDA survey found that peaches are the most pesticide-laden fruit in the produce section, so if you can afford organic, you might want to spring.

(Nutritional info is for a 1-cup serving, unless otherwise stated)

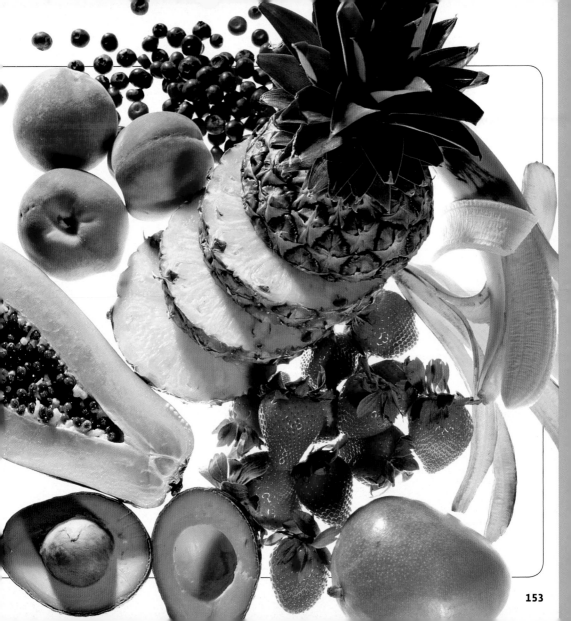

Liquids

Orange Juice

112 calories

0 g fat

21 g sugars

OJ's balance of sweetness and acidity makes it a versatile smoothie constituent, capable of tying together seemingly disparate fruit flavors. Even more of a conciliator are the orange juice blends, which usually incorporate juice from strawberries, pineapple, mango, or banana. Just make sure the label says 100 percent juice, otherwise you're paying for sugar water.

Pomegranate Juice

134 calories

0 g fat

32 g sugars

Pomegranates have been mythologized by everyone from the Greeks to Bible scribes, but the attention, at least from a nutritional standpoint, is not unwarranted. A study in the *American Journal of the College of Cardiology* found that 8 ounces of pomegranate juice a day increased blood flow to the heart. *The Journal of Urology* also found that 8 ounces of pomegranate juice a day

helped prostate cancer patients wean off their chemo and homone treatment.

And now there's a mounting body of evidence that pomegranate may help fight off cancer, in particular prostate and breast cancer. Don't be fooled by juice companies looking to capitalize on pomegranate's vaunted health reputation; many of them put only a drop of real pomegranate in their vats of cheap apple and grape juice. Make sure what you buy has just one ingredient: pomegranate.

1% Milk

102 calories

2 g fat
(2 g saturated)

13 g sugars

8 g protein

We love a splash of milk in our smoothies. Not only does it up the protein quotient, but it also brings about 30 percent of your day's calcium, vitamin D, and riboflavin to the glass. You're welcome to use skim, but some of milk's many nutrients are fat-soluble, meaning just a touch of dairy fat will help your body better absorb their benefits.

Soy Milk

132 calories

4.5 g fat
(0.5 g saturated)

10 g sugars

8 g protein

There's has been a long-running debate over the health benefits of soy. Most of that debate revolves around isoflavones, chemicals found in soy that are similar to estrogen. Some studies have found them to be beneficial in the fight against breast cancer, while others have found them to increase the likelihood of prostate cancer. While the researchers battle that one out, we can comfortably say that as a smoothie lubricator, soy milk will do just fine, especially for those unable to drink real milk. Unlike regular milk, soy milk won't give you the hit of calcium, but it will deliver a similar dose of protein.

Green Tea

0 calories

0 g fat

0 g sugars

Not a traditional smoothie liquid, but a damn fine one, especially if we're talking about unsweetened green tea. Add a half-cup or more and you'll not only get a hit of caffeine, but a big dose of

catechins, the antioxidants in green tea that are known to boost metabolism and help our bodies burn calories quicker.

Coffee

2 calories

0 g fat

0 g sugars

What could be more convenient than combining your morning buzz and your breakfast in a single glass? Especially when that buzz is such a tremendous superfood. A recent review of coffee research published in the *Archives of Internal Medicine* found that for every cup of coffee consumed daily you can lower your risk of type 2 diabetes by 7 percent. Add to that the abundance of antioxidants found in joe and you have a pretty convincing case to make coffee a go-to smoothie ingredient. Just make sure the coffee is cool, as no one wants a warm smoothie. It's also best if it's really strong, preferably espresso-strength, so that you don't water down your smoothie.

(Nutritional info is for a 1-cup serving, unless otherwise stated)

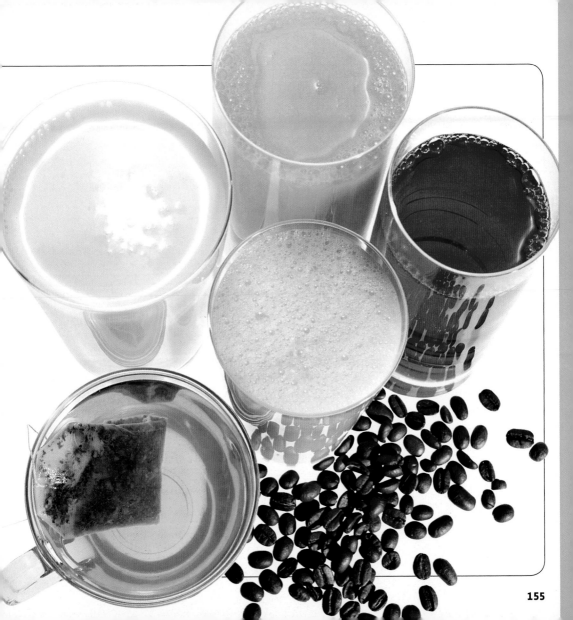

Thickeners & Enhancers

Peanut Butter
(1 Tbsp)

94 calories

8 g fat
(1.5 g saturated)

1 g sugars

3.5 g protein

What's not to love about peanut butter? The fat is good for your heart, the protein is good for your muscles, and the package of vitamins and nutrients (vitamin E, manganese, niacin) will do plenty for the rest of your body. The only drawback is that peanut butter is extremely dense with calories (and don't bother with the reduced fat stuff—it's loaded with chemicals), so try to keep the quantity to about half a tablespoon per smoothie.

Fat-Free Greek-Style Yogurt
(½ cup)

70 calories

0 g fat

5 g sugars

12 g protein

There may be no better addition to a smoothie than a healthy scoop of Greek yogurt. Not only does it give the smoothie a lovely body, but it also adds a ton of protein and gut-friendly bacteria to whatever

concoction it graces. Why Greek? Because the Greeks are savvy enough to skim off the watery whey found in typical yogurt, thus yielding a creamier product with more than twice the protein found in the Dannons and the Yoplaits of the dairy world. Both Fage and Oikos are reliable brands found in most supermarkets. If you must stick to regular American-style yogurt, just make sure it's unflavored; opt for a fruit- or vanilla-flavored yogurt and you might as well be using ice cream.

Honey
(1 Tbsp)

64 calories

0 g fat

17 g sugars

As far as sweeteners go, honey ranks high on the list for the simple fact that it actually gives you something in return for all that sugar, namely a host of phytonutrients that have antiviral and antibacterial properties. Still, added sugar in any form is highly discouraged in the craft of smoothie making, so use honey sparingly, if at all.

Fresh Mint/ Fresh Basil
(2 Tbsp)

2 calories

0 g fat

0 g sugars

Strange though it may sound, adding fresh herbs to smoothies is a small little trick that yields big results when properly employed. Plus, when you consider that fresh basil contains cancer-fighting carotenoids and that the menthol in mint can help facilitate easy breathing and relieve indigestion, what more motivation do you need? Basil pairs well with strawberries and watermelon, while mint works wonders on melon, blueberries, and papaya.

Agave Syrup
(1 Tbsp)

60 calories

0 g fat

15 g sugars

Let's be clear: As long as your smoothie is composed primarily of fruit, there is no reason to add sugar to the mix. But if you ever do reach for it, agave syrup is the way to go. The sweetness comes primarily from a form of fructose called inulin, which has a very gentle effect on your blood sugar, which not only helps

prevent the dreaded sugar crash, but also keeps your body from going into fat storage mode. Score a bottle at most health food stores and grocers like Whole Foods.

Fat-Free Frozen Yogurt
(½ cup)

100 calories

0 g fat

14 g sugars

Jamba Juice, Smoothie King, and other popular smoothie purveyors grab the fro-yo with regularity, but that doesn't mean you should. Just like there's no use for added sweeteners in a real smoothie, there's no place for a dessert-like scoop, either. The fact that frozen yogurt, like sherbet, is often fat free means nothing; the culprit is the 14 grams of sugar—nearly as much as you'd get from a pack of Reese's Peanut Butter Cups. Save this stuff for milk shakes.

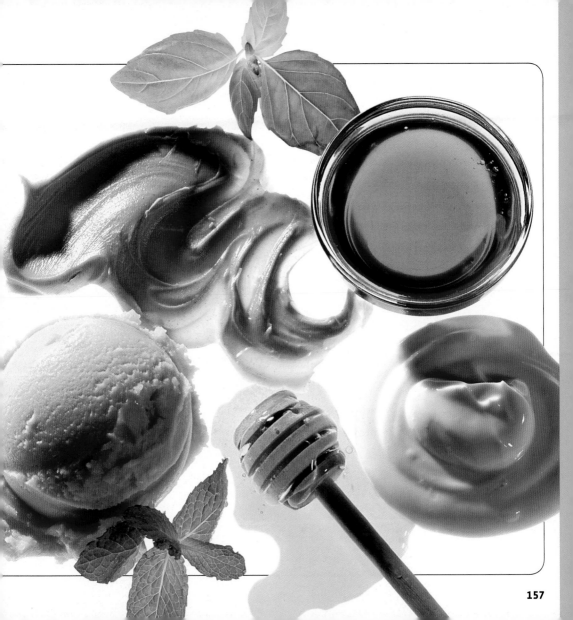

Boosts

Protein Powder
(2 Tbsp)

104 calories

0 g fat

16 g protein

No, protein powder isn't just for the muscle mag set. Dozens of studies have highlighted the importance of getting protein first thing in the morning. Not only will it help to jolt your metabolism into action, it's also been shown to help you retain focus throughout the morning.

Fiber Boost
(2 Tbsp)

35 calories

0 g fat

9 g fiber

Often sold under the name of psyllium husk (for the seeds this powder is ground from), a dose of fiber is going to do more than promote a healthy colon. Fiber will slow the digestion of the smoothie in your stomach, which not only means you'll stay fuller longer, but also that the sugar from the fruit will have a less dramatic impact on your blood sugar levels. And if the Quaker Oats dude has taught us anything, it's that fiber promotes a healthy heart, as well.

Fish Oil
(1 tsp)

41 calories

5 g fat
(1 g saturated)

1,084 mg omega-3s

Fish oil has been canonized by hoards of wide-eyed nutritionists over the years, but the case for its saint-hood sure is compelling. The tide of omega-3 fatty acids found in fish oil (usually made from fatty fish like salmon and sardines) may be the most versatile nutritional weapon out there, known to help protect the heart, fight inflammation, boost the brain, and reduce blood pressure, among other things. Look for a brand with a subtle flavor that will add all of the nutritional punch without leaving your smoothie tasting like a can of sardines. We like Carlson Fish Oil liquids.

Ground Flaxseed
(2 Tbsp)

80 calories

5 g fat
(1 g saturated)

2,700 mg omega-3s

These seeds, picked and ground from the flax plant commonly found across the Mediterranean and Middle East, deliver a mother lode of omega-3s. Consider stirring them into your oatmeal or yogurt, but if you're looking for the easiest way to sneak flax into your diet, look to the blender for seamless integration.

Multivitamin Powder
(1 packet/Tbsp)

0 calories

Great for kids, of course, but given how few adults are eating their fruits and vegetables, smoothie drinkers of all ages should embrace a multivitamin boost. You can pick your product based upon your specific needs, but expect a massive dose of two dozen or more essential nutrients. Pick up a box at a health food store and add it to the base of your smoothie.

Wheatgrass Powder
(1.25 Tbsp)

35 calories

What doesn't wheatgrass offer? Even a tiny dose like this packs fiber, protein, tons of vitamin A and K, folic acid, manganese, iodine, and chlrophyll, to name a few. You don't need to know what each nutrient does for you; just know that a single tablespoon will have you operating at peak perfor-mance levels. Pick some up at amazinggrass.com.

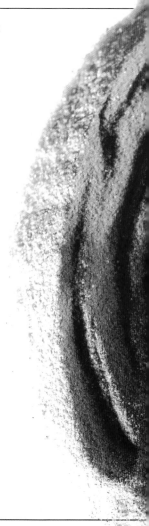

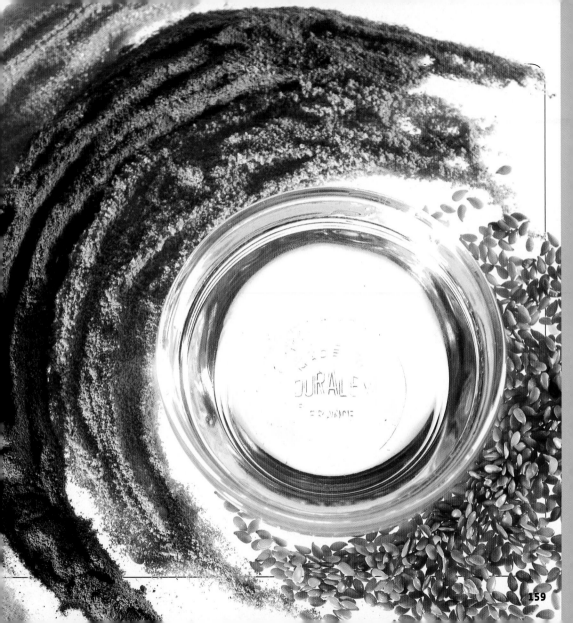

Smoothies

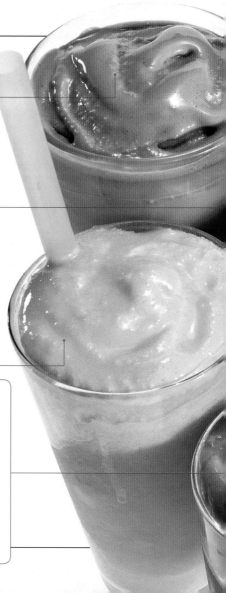

The Caffeinated Banana

1 very ripe banana
½ cup strong coffee
½ cup milk
1 Tbsp peanut butter
1 Tbsp agave syrup
1 cup ice

With protein, healthy fat, and caffeine, this works perfectly as a start to your day or as a low-cal substitute for a milk shake.

311 calories, 10 g fat, 38 g sugars

The Blue Monster

1 cup blueberries
½ cup pomegranate or blueberry juice
½ cup yogurt
3 or 4 cubes of ice
1 Tbsp flaxseed

Between the polyphenols in the blueberries and the pomegranate and the omega-3s in the flax, we're talking serious brain food.

258 calories, 4 g fat, 38 g sugars

The Orange Crush

¾ cup frozen mango
½ cup carrot juice
½ cup orange juice
½ cup Greek yogurt
1 Tbsp protein powder
½ cup water

All that orange produce means this baby is stuffed full of vision-strengthening, cancer-fighting carotenoids.

280 calories, 1 g fat, 38 g sugars

Papaya Berry

¾ cup frozen papaya
¾ cup frozen strawberries
½ cup milk
½ cup orange juice
1Tbsp fresh mint

This is like a liquid mulitvitamin, loaded with vitamins A and C, plus disease-fighting carotenoids and lycopene.

188 calories, 2 g fat, 28 g sugars

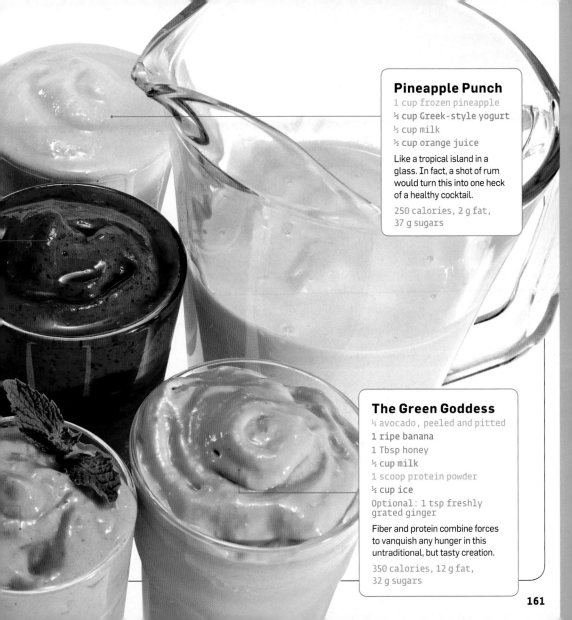

Pineapple Punch

1 cup frozen pineapple
½ cup Greek-style yogurt
½ cup milk
½ cup orange juice

Like a tropical island in a glass. In fact, a shot of rum would turn this into one heck of a healthy cocktail.

250 calories, 2 g fat, 37 g sugars

The Green Goddess

¼ avocado, peeled and pitted
1 ripe banana
1 Tbsp honey
½ cup milk
1 scoop protein powder
½ cup ice

Optional: 1 tsp freshly grated ginger

Fiber and protein combine forces to vanquish any hunger in this untraditional, but tasty creation.

350 calories, 12 g fat, 32 g sugars

JAMBA JUICE

● We love smoothies as much as anyone, but they're not always the magic bullet that some would like to believe. And what's more, those who mistakenly order one of Jamba's surreptitious sugar bombs might be unwittingly sabotaging their waistline. That said, there are plenty of first-rate all-fruit blends to satisfy even the pickiest palate that offer up a quick, definitive solution to the enduring lack of produce in the American diet. And Jamba's recent expansion of its food options, including a strong line of oatmeals and flatbreads, only deepens the diversity of an already-solid menu.

Drink This

Strawberry Whirl

with Whey Protein Super Boost (small, 16 fl oz)

265 calories
0 g fat
46 g sugars

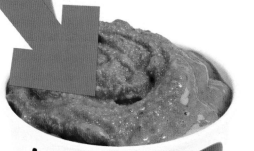

A whey boost is the easiest way to transform a light snack into a light meal. For 45 calories you get 10 grams of protein, enough to keep you full longer and help regulate the post-smoothie blood-sugar flux.

Other Picks

Perfectly Chocolate Chai Tea Latte with 2% Milk
(small, 16 fl oz)
280 calories
6 g fat
(3.5 g saturated)
41 g sugars

Berry Fulfilling
(power size, 30 fl oz)
320 calories
1 g fat
(0 g saturated)
53 g sugars

Bright Eyed and Blueberry
(small, 16 fl oz)
240 calories
0 g fat
40 g sugars

570 calories
17 g fat
(2.5 g saturated)
54 g sugars

Not That!

Ideal Meal Chunky Strawberry

(small, 16 fl oz)

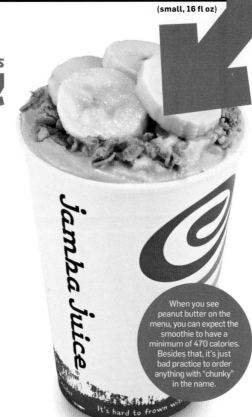

Other Passes

Chill-icious Chai
(original size, 22 fl oz)
440 calories
0 g fat
82 g sugars

Razzmatazz
(power size, 30 fl oz)
520 calories
2.5 g fat
(1 g saturated)
100 g sugars

Berry Topper
(small, 16 fl oz)
480 calories
9 g fat
(1.5 g saturated)
55 g sugars

When you see peanut butter on the menu, you can expect the smoothie to have a minimum of 470 calories. Besides that, it's just bad practice to order anything with "chunky" in the name.

For 570 calories, you can have

ALL THIS

A MediterraneYUM California Flatbread, an Omega-3 Chocolate Brownie Cookie, and a 12-ounce Cup of Orange Juice

OR

THAT

A Chocolate Moo'd
(original size, 22 fl oz)

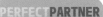

PERFECT PARTNER

Fresh Banana Oatmeal
280 calories
4 g fat (1 g saturated)
19 g sugars

This isn't your grocery store's instant oatmeal. Jamba's are slow-cooked steel-cut oats, prepared with creamy soy milk and topped with real fruit. Pair a cup with a small juice or smoothie for a near-perfect breakfast packed with protein and fiber.

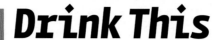

Drink This

Mango Mantra

(original size, 22 fl oz)

250 calories
1 g fat
(0 g saturated)
48 g sugars

STEALTH HEALTH FOOD
Bananas

Sure each banana has 15 to 20 grams of sugar, but that's a perfect load for the base of a naturally sweetened beverage. Plus it comes with powerhouse prebiotics inulin and oligofructose. The first is a powerful fiber, and the second is a sugar that nurtures the bacteria that keep your stomach healthy.

Other Picks

Protein Berry Workout with Whey

(original size, 22 oz)
370 calories
0.5 g fat
59 g sugars
20 g protein

Orange Carrot Banana Juice

(small, 16 fl oz)
170 calories
1 g fat
26 g sugars

The Mantra comes from Jamba's light menu, which means it's made with a low-calorie dairy base consisting of milk and Splenda. If you'd like to nix the sweetener, try the Mega Mango on the always-dependable All Fruit menu. The original size has 320 calories.

Strawberry Nirvana

(original size, 22 fl oz)
230 calories
0.5 g fat
(0 g saturated)
43 g sugars

It's hard to frown with a straw

400 calories
1.5 g fat
(0.5 g saturated)
85 g sugars

Not That!

Mango-a-Go-Go

(original size, 22 fl oz)

ALL STAR ADDITIVES

3G Charger
5 calories

An antioxidant-loaded blend of inulin, green tea and guarana extracts, and ginseng root. Plus it's fortified with 2 grams of fiber.

Flax and Fiber Boost
30 calories

Imparts a massive 7 grams of fiber, mostly from flaxseed, which is also the source of the healthy omega-3 fats.

Whey Protein
45 calories

This dairy-based additive adds 10 grams of protein and the essential amino acids your body needs to function. Perfect for a post-workout snack.

Energy Boost
0 calories

Forget the canned energy drinks; this boost gives your smoothie the same stuff: a dose of taurine and a massive supply of energy-inducing B vitamins.

Other Passes

Peanut Butter M'ood
(original size, 22 oz)
770 calories
20 g fat
(4.5 g saturated)
108 g sugars
20 g protein

Orange Juice
(small, 16 fl oz)
220 calories
1 g fat
42 g sugars

Strawberry Energizer
(original size, 22 fl oz)
390 calories
1.5 g fat
(0.5 g saturated)
82 g sugars

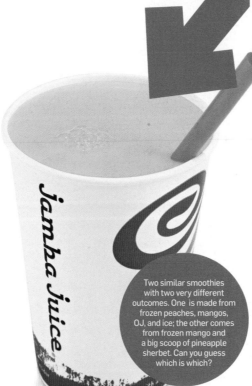

Two similar smoothies with two very different outcomes. One is made from frozen peaches, mangos, OJ, and ice; the other comes from frozen mango and a big scoop of pineapple sherbet. Can you guess which is which?

SMOOTHIE KING

● Why does Smoothie King score so much worse than Jamba Juice? Portion Distortion. Consider this: A true beverage serving is 8 fluid ounces. At Smoothie King, even the small is 20. A large is 40, which is the equivalent of five normal servings. That's how the calories stack up so quickly (Smoothie King has 32 drinks with more than 1,000 calories). Here's the upside: You can request any smoothie be prepared without added sugars. Just ask for it in a small cup.

FOOD COURT

THE CRIME
32-ounce Banana Boat Smoothie
(825 calories)

THE PUNISHMENT
2 hours chopping wood

Drink This

The Strawberry Shredder
(small, 20 fl oz)

356 calories
1 g fat
(0 g saturated)
41 g sugars

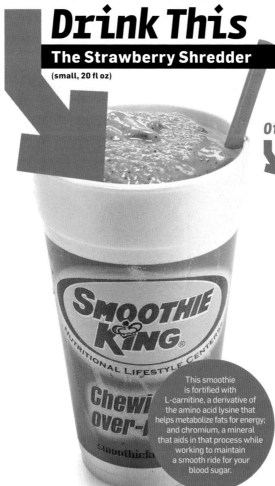

This smoothie is fortified with L-carnitine, a derivative of the amino acid lysine that helps metabolize fats for energy; and chromium, a mineral that aids in that process while working to maintain a smooth ride for your blood sugar.

Other Picks

High Protein Almond Mocha
(small, 20 fl oz)
366 calories
9 g fat
(1 g saturated)
37 g sugars

Youth Fountain
(small, 20 fl oz)
253 calories
0 g fat
54 g sugars

Skinny Coconut Surprise
(small, 20 fl oz)
260 calories
7 g fat
(6 g saturated)
37 g sugars

712 calories
25 g fat
(6 g saturated)
94 g sugars

Not That!
Strawberry Peanut Power Plus
(small, 20 fl oz)

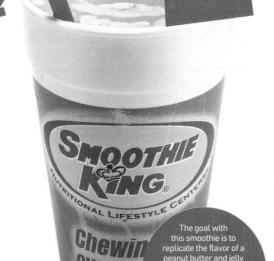

Other Passes

The Hulk Chocolate
(small, 20 fl oz)
905 calories
35 g fat
(16 g saturated)
88 g sugars

Light and Fluffy
(small, 20 fl oz)
395 calories
0 g fat
89 g sugars

Skinny Piña Colada Island
(small, 20 fl oz)
400 calories
10 g fat
(8 g saturated)
52 g sugars

The goal with this smoothie is to replicate the flavor of a peanut butter and jelly sandwich. That would be fine if it weren't for the fact that Smoothie King's PB&J comes laced with 200 calories of added sugar.

WEAPON OF MASS DESTRUCTION
The Hulk Strawberry
(large, 40 fl oz)

2,088 calories
70 g fat (32 g saturated)
240 g sugars

Allow us to introduce you to the most caloric drink in America. It's made with butter pecan ice cream, egg protein, and a "carbohydrate mix" that probably consists of mostly sugar. If you're really looking to put on weight, there are less catastrophic ways of doing it.

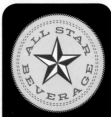

Berry Stimulating Mate (small, 20 fl oz)

348 calories
0 g fat
81 g sugars

Mate, an Argentinean herb, has been shown to have as much as 90 percent more metabolism-boosting polyphenols than green tea. Blending it with blueberries, blackberries, and strawberries resulted in one of the most nutritionally potent beverages in America.

Drink This

Pineapple Pleasure

(small, 20 fl oz)

280 calories
0 g fat
61 g sugars

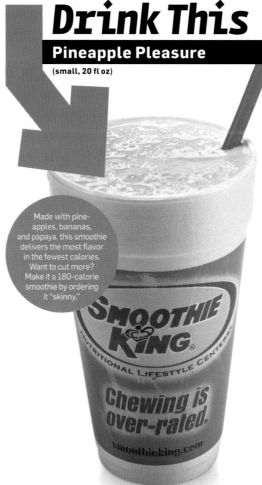

Made with pineapples, bananas, and papaya, this smoothie delivers the most flavor in the fewest calories. Want to cut more? Make it a 180-calorie smoothie by ordering it "skinny."

Other Picks

Blueberry Heaven
(small, 20 fl oz)
325 calories
1 g fat
(0 g saturated)
64 g sugars

Muscle Punch Plus
(small, 20 fl oz)
366 calories
1 g fat
(0 g saturated)
75 g sugars

Yerba Maté Pomegranate
(small, 20 fl oz)
372 calories
0 g fat
73 g sugars

SIZE MATTERS!

CRANBERRY COOLER

LARGE

(40 fl oz)
992 calories

CRANBERRY COOLER

small

(20 fl oz)
496 calories

**Total Savings:
496 CALORIES!**

461 calories
1 g fat
(0 g saturated)
92 g sugars

Not That!

Pineapple Surf

(small, 20 fl oz)

Other Passes

Grape Expectations II
(small, 20 fl oz)
548 calories
0 g fat
125 g sugars

Power Punch Plus
(small, 20 fl oz)
500 calories
1 g fat
(0 g saturated)
85 g sugars

Cranberry Supreme
(small, 20 fl oz)
554 calories
1 g fat
(0 g saturated)
96 g sugars

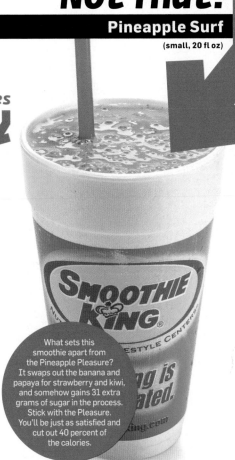

What sets this smoothie apart from the Pineapple Pleasure? It swaps out the banana and papaya for strawberry and kiwi, and somehow gains 31 extra grams of sugar in the process. Stick with the Pleasure. You'll be just as satisfied and cut out 40 percent of the calories.

SUGAR SPIKE

Grape Expectations II
(large, 40 fl oz)

The Impact:
250 GRAMS!

Grape juice contains more sugar than orange, apple, pineapple, or any other common contender, which is why it's a bad choice as the base of a smoothie. Especially when you blend it with even more sugar. The result is a beverage with nearly as much sugar as an entire 2-liter bottle of grape soda.

GUILTY PLEASURE

Coffee Mocha
(small, 20 fl oz)

260 calories
2 g fat (0 g saturated)
36 g sugars

Even better than being simply low in calories and sugar (especially compared to coffee-shop mochas) is the fact that it's also high in protein—a 20-ounce cup has 17 grams.

Drink This

Your goal: Buy only 100% juice or "light" juice free of added sugars.

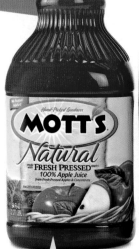

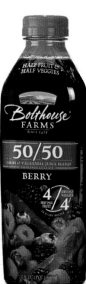

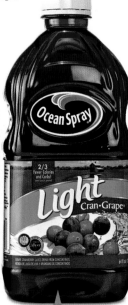

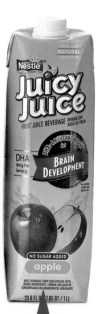

Mott's Natural 100% Apple Juice
(8 fl oz)

110 calories
0 g fat
27 g sugars

In the battle of apple versus grape, apple comes out the caloric winner every time.

Bolthouse Farms 50/50 Berry
(8 fl oz)

120 calories
0 g fat
28 g sugars

Vegetable-fruit blends make for excellent juices. This one contains a huge antioxidant kick from purple carrots, blackberries, pomegranates, and blueberries.

Ocean Spray Light Cran-Grape
(8 fl oz)

40 calories
0 g fat
10 g sugars

Ocean Spray's light line of cranberry blends actually boasts a higher percentage of real juice than the regular line. Here, light earns you 10% more juice for 80 fewer calories.

Juicy Juice Brain Development Apple
(8 fl oz)

80 calories
0 g fat
18 g sugars

The addition of brain-boosting fish oil is good, but the real genius of this juice is that it uses a splash of water to cut down on the sugar.

Not That!

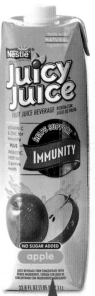

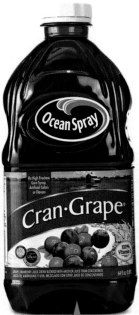

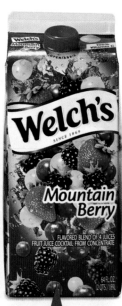

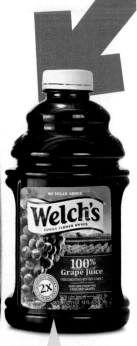

Juicy Juice Immunity Apple (8 fl oz)

100 calories
0 g fat
18 g sugars

Sure, zinc is good for the immune system, but the amount in this juice is about as much as you'd get from an ounce of red meat or a half cup of yogurt.

Ocean Spray Cran-Grape (8 fl oz)

120 calories
0 g fat
31 g sugars

Ocean Spray is notorious for polluting their juices with high-fructose corn syrup. This particular bottle has just 15% juice, meaning the other 85% is colored sugar water.

Welch's Mountain Berry (8 fl oz)

140 calories
0 g fat
33 g sugars

For this many calories, you should expect nothing less than 100% juice. This one falls short with only 25%.

Welch's 100% Grape Juice (8 fl oz)

160 calories
0 g fat
39 g sugars

Yes, grape juice offers some of the same heart-healthy benefits as wine, but it's also the most sugar-loaded juice on the shelves. We'll take the wine and skip the juice.

Drink This

*Whether or not it's made from 100% juice,
if your bottle packs more than 120 calories per serving,
put it back on the shelf.*

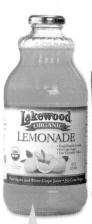

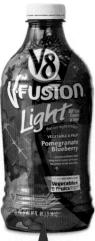

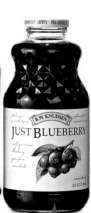

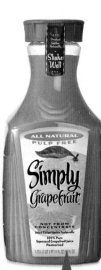

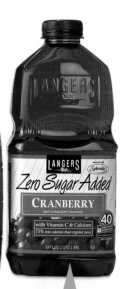

Lakewood Organic Lemonade
(8 fl oz)

86 calories
0 g fat
19 g sugars

Instead of sugar, this bottle is sweetened with grape juice and agave nectar. As good as lemonade gets.

V-Fusion Light Pomegranate Blueberry
(8 fl oz)

50 calories
0 g fat
10 g sugars

Every calorie in this bottle comes from the blend of sweet potatoes, carrots, apples, pomegranates, and blueberries.

R.W. Knudsen Just Blueberry
(8 fl oz)

100 calories
0 g fat
18 g sugars

Blueberries are bursting with brain-boosting antioxidants, and R.W. Knudsen's juice is the only one to give you 100% blueberries.

Simply Grapefruit
(8 fl oz)

90 calories
0 g fat
18 g sugars

Grapefruit is the most underrated juice in the cooler. It's delicious, it's naturally low in sugar, and it delivers a dose of cancer-fighting lycopene.

Langers Zero Sugar Added Cranberry
(8 fl oz)

30 calories
0 g fat
8 g sugars

Cranberries make for a tart juice, which is why you routinely see 15 or more grams of sugar added to each serving.

Not That!

Limit juice consumption to just 8 ounces a day. The rest of your fruit and vegetable intake should be coming from the real stuff.

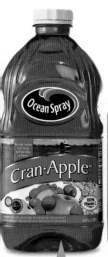

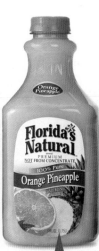

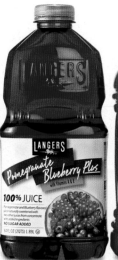

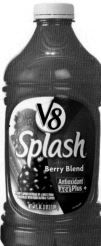

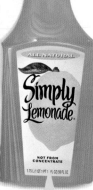

Ocean Spray Cran-Apple
(8 fl oz)

130 calories
0 g fat
32 g sugars

This bottle, like so many in Ocean Spray's lineup, contains only 15% juice. Water and sugar are the first two ingredients.

Florida's Natural 100% Pure Orange Pineapple
(8 fl oz)

130 calories
0 g fat
30 g sugars

It's hard to fault 100% juice products, but blends like this tend to pack in too much sugar.

Langers Pomegranate Blueberry Plus
(8 fl oz)

140 calories
0 g fat
32 g sugars

There's more sugar in this bottle than there are blueberries or pomegranates.

V8 Splash Berry Blend
(8 fl oz)

70 calories
0 g fat
18 g sugars

Splash is unfit to carry the V8 brand name. It's made with artificial colors, high-fructose corn syrup, and a pathetic 10% juice.

Simply Lemonade
(8 fl oz)

120 calories
0 g fat
28 g sugars

Contains only 11% juice. The rest of the bottle is pure sugar water. Most lemonades follow the same disappointing formula.

173

SMOOTHIES

Drink This

You're always best off blending your own smoothies, but when in a pinch, the ones below will do the trick.

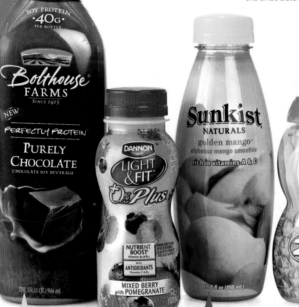

Bolthouse Farms Perfectly Protein Purely Chocolate
(15.2 fl oz bottle)

323 calories
4.5 g fat
(0 g saturated)
38 g sugars

Protein drinks tend to be high in calories. This is one of the best you'll find.

Dannon Light and Fit 0% Fat Plus Mixed Berry Pomegranate
(7 fl oz bottle)

70 calories
0 g fat
12 g sugars

You get more than double the drink, plus gut-friendly bacteria, for fewer calories.

Sunkist Naturals Golden Mango Smoothie
(15.2 fl oz bottle)

266 calories
0 g fat
49.5 g sugars

The sugar is 100% natural, and it comes packed with nearly 6 grams of fiber to help ease it into your blood.

Fruit2day Pineapple Banana
(6.75 fl oz bottle)

120 calories
0 g fat
22 g sugars

A relatively low-calorie snack with real pineapple chunks in the bottle.

Not That!

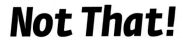

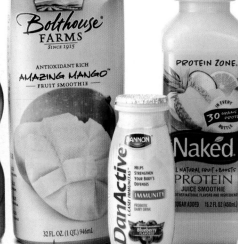

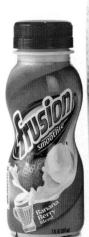

Frusion Smoothie Banana Berry Blend
(7 fl oz)

180 calories
2.5 g fat
(1.5 g saturated)
33 g sugars

Look for smoothies sweetened with honey or agave syrup. The high-fructose corn syrup in this bottle just won't cut it.

Bolthouse Farms Amazing Mango
(15.2 fl oz bottle)

323 calories
0 g fat
60 g sugars

If your smoothie has more than 300 calories, it officially counts as a meal.

Dannon DanActive Blueberry
(3.1 fl oz bottle)

80 calories
1.5 g fat
(1 g saturated)
13 g sugars

More than twice as calorie-dense as a can of Mountain Dew.

Naked Protein Juice Smoothie
(15.2 fl oz)

418 calories
3.5 g fat
(2 g saturated)
53 g sugars

At 31 grams, this is one of the most protein-rich smoothies on the market. Too bad it's also one of the most caloric.

Drink This

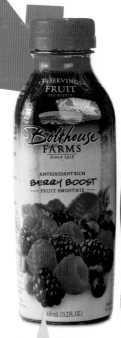

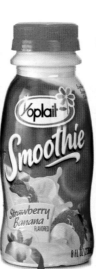

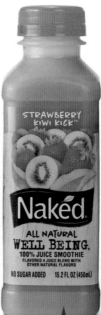

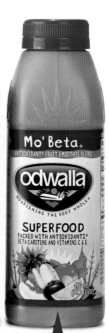

**Bolthouse Farms
Berry Boost
(15.2 fl oz bottle)**

209 calories
0 g fat
49.5 g sugars

This bottle has nearly
8 grams of fiber—that's
just under a third of
your daily intake.

**Yoplait
Strawberry
Banana Smoothie
(about 8 fl oz prepared
with skim milk)**

110 calories
1.5 g fat
(1 g saturated)
16.5 g sugars

The easiest 50 calories
you'll ever save.

**Naked
Strawberry
Kiwi Kick
(15.2 fl oz bottle)**

209 calories
0 g fat
44 g sugars

At this size, you
won't find a smoothie
with fewer calories.

**Odwalla Mo' Beta
Superfood
(15.2 fl oz bottle)**

228 calories
0 g fat
42 g sugars

This is the lightest of the
so-called superfood
smoothies. Plus, it arms
your immune system with
about 2 days' worth of
vitamin A and 6 days
of vitamin E.

Not That!

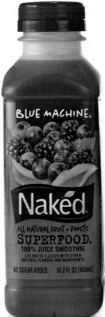

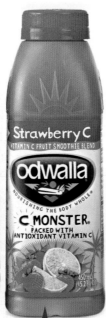

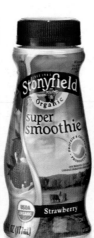

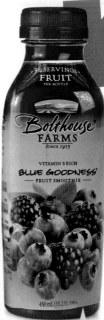

**Naked Blue
Machine
Superfood**
(15.2 fl oz bottle)

323 calories
0 g fat
55 g sugars

This shake performs well
nutritionally, but
unfortunately it carries
too much sugar to be
considered a wise choice.

**Odwalla
Strawberry C
Monster**
(15.2 fl oz bottle)

304 calories
0 g fat
55 g sugars

We're impressed this
bottle carries 2,900%
of your daily vitamin C.
We'd be even more
impressed if it carried
less sugar.

**Stonyfield Farm
Organic Smoothie
Strawberry**
(6 fl oz bottle)

140 calories
2 g fat
(1 g saturated)
23 g sugars

Dear Stonyfield, we love
the organic yogurt,
but please cut the sugar
in half. Sincerely,
Eat This, Not That.

**Bolthouse Farms
Blue Goodness**
(15.2 fl oz bottle)

323 calories
0 g fat
53 g sugars

Loaded with fiber, but
also loaded with calories.
You want a smoothie
that can balance the two.

SINGLE-SERVING JUICES

Drink This

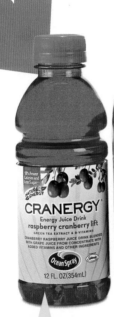

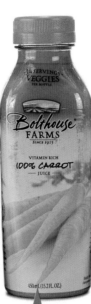

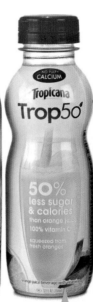

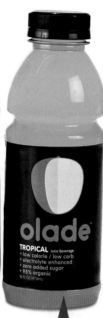

Ocean Spray Cranergy Raspberry Cranberry Lift
(12 fl oz bottle)

50 calories
0 g fat
13 g sugars

This low-cal juice blend packs an impressive package of energy-inducing B vitamins.

Bolthouse Farms 100% Carrot Juice
(15.2 fl oz bottle)

140 calories
0 g fat
28 g sugars

Low in calories and sugar and laced with 700% of your daily vitamin A. If you don't like the taste of straight carrot, cut it with a touch of 100% OJ.

Tropicana Trop50
(12 fl oz bottle)

80 calories
0 g fat
15 g sugars

By cutting the OJ with water without adding additional sugar, Tropicana has created a juice drink that's low enough in calories to drink every day.

Olade Tropical Juice Beverage
(16 fl oz bottle)

20 calories
0 g fat
4 g sugars

This bottle manages the calories by supplementing a 20% blend of lemon, pineapple, mango, and passion fruit juices with the non-caloric stevia extract.

Be wary of all individual "juice" products. Many of them are merely soft drinks in disguise.

ot That!

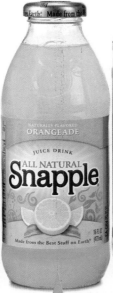

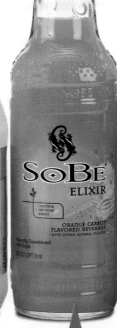

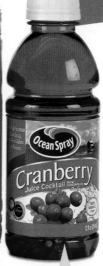

Sunny D Tangy Original
(6.75 fl oz bottle)

80 calories
0 g fat
16 g sugars

With only 5% juice, Sunny D would be better thought of as a noncarbonated soda.

Snapple Orangeade
(16 fl oz bottle)

200 calories
0 g fat
52 g sugars

The suffix "-ade" is your clue that this bottle is loaded with high-fructose corn syrup.

SoBe Elixir Orange Carrot
(20 fl oz bottle)

220 calories
0 g fat
56 g sugars

Both oranges and carrots play a supporting role. The real star, as with all of SoBe's Elixirs, is sugar.

Ocean Spray Cranberry Juice Cocktail
(12 fl oz bottle)

180 calories
0 g fat
45 g sugars

Avoid juice "cocktails" at all costs; here it means just 27% juice. Turn to Cranergy instead—our favorite Ocean Spray product.

Drink This

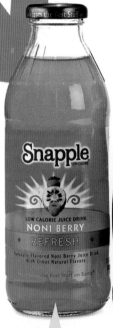

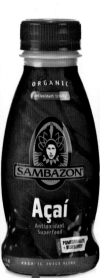

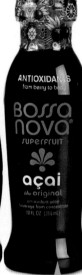

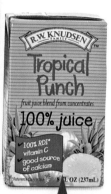

Snapple Noni Berry Refresh
(17.5 fl oz bottle)

30 calories
0 g fat
3 g sugars

Snapple isn't a juice company, as most of their bottles contain 10% or less of the real stuff. But this ranks among their best products.

Sambazon Antioxidant Trinity Açai with Pomegranate and Blueberry
(10.5 fl oz)

143 calories
0 g fat
27 g sugars

High in calories, but it packs a roster of the world's most nutrient-rich fruit.

Bossa Nova Açai
(10 fl oz bottle)

114 calories
0 g fat
22.5 g sugars

Some studies have found the Amazonian açai berry to have 700% more antioxidants than blueberries, often considered the most antioxidant-packed fruit.

R.W. Knudsen Tropical Punch
(8 fl oz box)

120 calories
0 g fat
27 g sugars

This box contains a 100% blend of apple, cherry, and raspberry juices. Just another reason why Knudsen is one of our favorite producers in the juice aisle.

Not That!

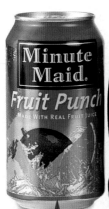
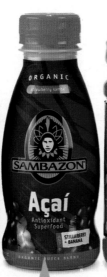
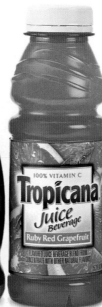
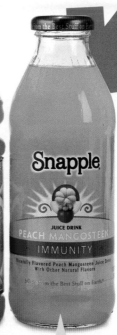

Minute Maid Fruit Punch
(12 fl oz can)

160 calories
0 g fat
43 g sugars

About 90% of the time, "fruit punch" means loads of sugar with a mere touch of juice. In this case, that touch accounts for a paltry 3% of the calories in this can.

Sambazon Açaí Strawberry Banana
(10.5 fl oz bottle)

208 calories
4 g fat
(0.5 g saturated)
39 g sugars

The wrong Sambazon juice blend will cost you. This one has 45% more calories than the one on the opposite page.

Tropicana Juice Beverage Ruby Red Grapefruit
(15.2 fl oz bottle)

250 calories
0 g fat
55 g sugars

Tropicana is sneaky with its juice line. The 100% juice bottles and the ones loaded with HFCS are nearly indistinguishable. This, sadly, is the latter.

Snapple Peach Mangosteen Immunity
(17.5 fl oz bottle)

190 calories
0 g fat
44 g sugars

Sugar is the second ingredient. Since when have blood sugar spikes been proven to boost immunity?

KIDS' DRINKS

Drink This

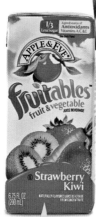

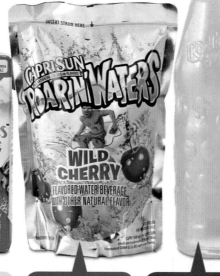

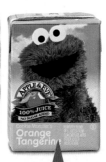

Apple & Eve Fruitables Fruit and Vegetable Strawberry Kiwi
(6.75 fl oz box)

70 calories
0 g fat
15 g sugars

Made from nine different fruits and vegetables without any added sugar.

Capri Sun Roarin' Waters Wild Cherry
(6 fl oz pouch)

30 calories
0 g fat
8 g sugars

If you're going to go with a nonjuice drink, it better at least be low in calories. This is a big improvement on Capri Sun's normal line of pouches.

Kool-Aid Bursts Grape
(6.75 fl oz bottle)

35 calories
0 g fat
9 g sugars

For once Kool-Aid decides to go light on the sugar. Other than that, there's nothing particularly redeeming about this bottle.

Apple and Eve Cookie Monster's Orange Tangerine
(4.23 fl oz box)

60 calories
0 g fat
14 g sugars

This juice bucks the trend of using TV personalities to sell junk food to kids. This one is a 100% blend of tangerine, passion fruit, and pear juices.

Not That!

Kids' drink options have come a long way in recent years. Take advantage by picking a real 100% juice drink, or opting for one of the many new water-based beverages.

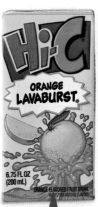

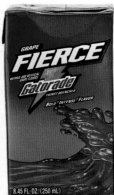

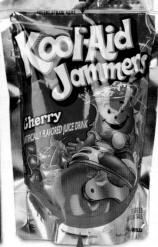

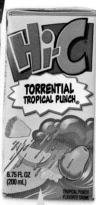

Hi-C Orange Lavaburst
(6.75 fl oz box)

90 calories
0 g fat
25 g sugars

The box might be bigger than Apple and Eve's but it actually packs less than 1 fluid ounce of real juice. Think about that the next time you're value shopping.

Gatorade Fierce Grape
(8.45 fl oz box)

60 calories
0 g fat
15 g sugars

Don't let the juice box fool you into thinking this is anything more than Gatorade's usual sugar-and-water formula.

Kool-Aid Jammers Cherry
(6 fl oz pouch)

80 calories
0 g fat
20 g sugars

The 5% juice in this bottle isn't even from cherries. It's pear juice. Never underestimate the twisted logic of the industrial food system.

Hi-C Torrential Tropical Punch
(6.75 fl oz box)

100 calories
0 g fat
25 g sugars

"Made with real fruit juice," as used on the front of this box, means 10% juice mixed with 90% water and high-fructose corn syrup.

Drink This

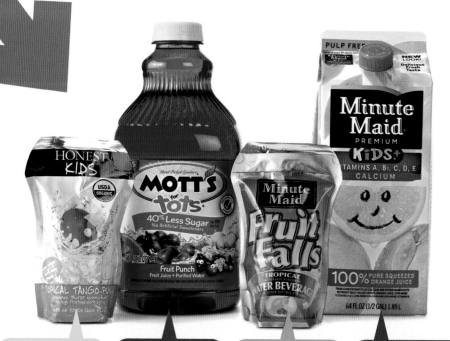

Honest Kids Tropical Tango Punch
(6.75 fl oz pouch)
40 calories
0 g fat
10 g sugars

Sweetened with fruit juice concentrates and fortified with 100% of your kid's daily vitamin C, plus a dose of added carotene.

Motts for Tots Fruit Punch
(8 fl oz)
60 calories
0 g fat
15 g sugars

This is an exceptional low-calorie juice for tots and adults alike. It's just juice and water.

Minute Maid Fruit Falls Tropical Water Beverage
(6.75 fl oz pouch)
5 calories
0 g fat
< 1 g sugars

Opt for a smaller portion and you can cap the sugar rush while still feeding your child real juice.

Minute Maid Kids+ Orange Juice
(8 fl oz)
110 calories
0 g fat
24 g sugars

This 100% juice is fortified with calcium and vitamins E and D. Perfect for growing bodies.

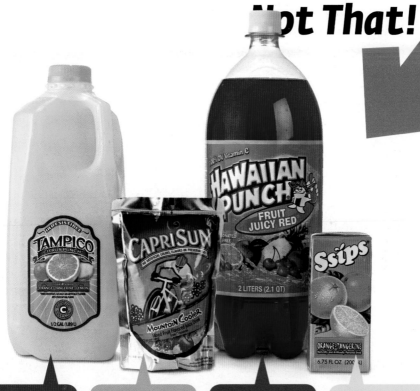

Not That!

Tampico Citrus Punch
(8 fl oz)

110 calories
0 g fat
27 g sugars

With less than 1% real juice, this is probably the worst kids' drink in the supermarket.

Capri Sun Mountain Cooler "25% less sugar"
(6 fl oz pouch)

60 calories
0 g fat
16 g sugars

We applaud Capri Sun for cutting back on the sugar, but the fact still remains: This is a high-calorie beverage containing just 10% juice.

Hawaiian Punch Fruit Juicy Red
(8 fl oz)

90 calories
0 g fat
22 g sugars

If you're going to give your kid the calories, you should also give her the nutrients. That means choosing real juice over juice imitators like this.

Ssips Orange-Tangerine
(6.75 fl oz box)

120 calories
0 g fat
30 g sugars

Made with just 10% juice and nearly twice as much sugar per ounce as you'd find in a can of Coke.

SPARKLING JUICE

Drink This

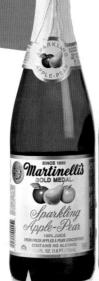
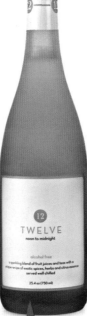
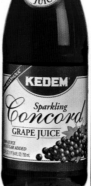
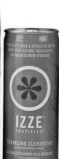
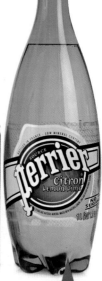

Martinelli's Sparkling Apple-Pear
(8 fl oz)

120 calories
0 g fat
24 g sugars

This is the best of Martinelli's array of sparklers: 100% apple juice mixed with pear concentrate.

Twelve
(8 fl oz)

60 calories
0 g fat
13 g sugars

Made from pineapple, grape, and peach juices, plus black and white teas and fresh herbs and spices. Delicous. Score a bottle at www.twelvebeverage.com.

Kedem Sparkling Concord Grape
(8 fl oz)

140 calories
0 g fat
35 g sugars

The fact that this is 100% juice makes it a perfect substitute for grape soda.

Izze Sparkling Clementine
(8.4 fl oz can)

90 calories
0 g fat
19 g sugars

Izze is a 70-30 blend of real juice and sparkling water. That leaves no room for added sugars.

Perrier Citron Lemon Lime
(22 fl oz bottle)

0 calories
0 g fat
0 g sugars

Want the bubbly without the bulge? Learn to love naturally scented, unsweetened sparkling waters.

Expect as much from your bubbly as you do your regular juice. Namely, as much fruit for as little sugar as possible.

Not That!

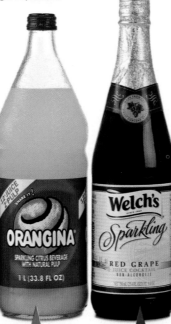

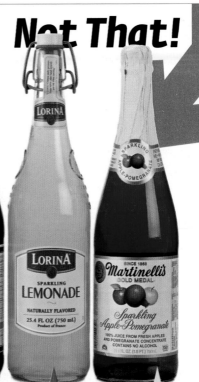

San Pellegrino Limonata
(11.15 fl oz can)

141 calories
0 g fat
32 g sugars

Don't be fooled by the fruit on the can. You'll find more calories inside than you'd get from the same size serving of Coke.

Orangina Sparkling Citrus Beverage
(8 fl oz)

100 calories
0 g fat
26 g sugars

Orangina contains just 12% juice. The rest of the sugar comes from HFCS.

Welch's Sparkling Red Grape Juice Cocktail
(8 fl oz)

160 calories
0 g fat
38 g sugars

Only 50% juice, which means the other 50% is water polluted with corn syrup.

Lorina Sparkling Lemonade
(8 fl oz)

90 calories
0 g fat
22 g sugars

Do you really want to pay a premium for gussied-up soda? The first two ingredients in this bottle are sugar and water.

Martinelli's Sparkling Apple-Pomegranate
(8 fl oz)

150 calories
0 g fat
32 g sugars

Pomegranate is found in more and more blends these days. Rarely are they good.

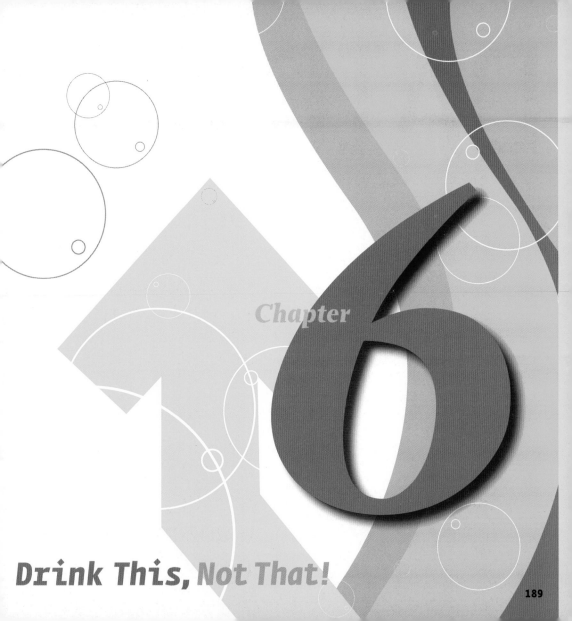

6

Drink This, Not That!

DAIRY

Quick Question: Do you want to lose weight, build lean muscle, have more energy, live longer, and protect yourself from heart disease, cancer, diabetes, stroke, and about a dozen other nasty diseases?

CHAPTER 6

Do you want to gain all those benefits and more—without ever exercising or dieting? And do you want to achieve all of those things in just 15 seconds a day, for less than 20 cents? No? Really? What's wrong with you?

Okay, let's just assume you answered yes. If so, we're going to teach you a simple habit that is going to change your life completely, making you slimmer, healthier, and more energetic all day long: Every morning when you get up out of bed, go stagger into the kitchen and fumble for your coffee mug—just like you do already. But don't pour coffee in it just yet. Instead, go directly to the fridge. Grab some low-fat milk. Fill the coffee cup with it. Drink that milk down to the point where there's the right amount left for your morning coffee. Now, add the coffee.

You've just started your day with one of the most effective weight-loss strategies known to man.

Seems crazy, but the perks of adopting that little habit are mind-blowing. First, you guarantee yourself the metabolism-boosting, energy-charging, hunger-suppressing, fat-burning, muscle-maintaining benefits of a high-protein breakfast—even if you don't get a chance to eat breakfast. (And you should still eat breakfast if you can—you want about 500 calories to start your day, and a cup of 2 percent milk has only 137.) Second, you guarantee you're getting at least 300 milligrams of calcium—almost half of the daily calcium amount shown to fend off weight gain, according to a Purdue University study. (In the study, women who took in at least 780 milligrams of calcium a day maintained their weight over a 2-year period, regardless of their exercise habits.

191

But women who took in less than that gained weight—again, regardless of whether they exercised or not!)

And if that's not enough to make you want to go hug a cow, consider this: Research shows that consuming calcium through dairy foods such as milk, yogurt, and cheese may also reduce fat absorption from other foods. In other words, drinking a glass of milk before you sit down to a giant, throbbing steak could actually trick your body into absorbing less of the steak's fat!

Now all of that is pretty exciting stuff. But even if you don't adopt our little morning ritual, drinking milk and noshing on other dairy products every day makes a lot of sense. The USDA recommends that adults ages 19 to 50 get at least 1,000 milligrams of calcium a day, and teens and those over 50 should get at least 1,300. But hitting those numbers is tough. Fortified cereals are the best source, but many of them are also loaded with sugar. Beyond that, your best nondairy sources of calcium are the tasty twofer of sardines and tofu— mmmm! Salmon, spinach, and collard greens also have healthy helpings, but few other foods even reach 100 milligrams per serving.

So yeah, milk is a great start. But there's a way you can take the benefits of milk up another notch or two: Spend just a little bit more and buy organic milk. Why? Because the nutrients in milk come from the nutrients that cows eat, and organic, pasture-raised cows eat healthier diets, meaning they create healthier milk. Recent studies revealed that organic dairy contains 75 percent more beta carotene, 70 percent more omega-3 fatty acids (the stuff in those expensive fish-oil supplements), and 50 percent more vitamin E than regular milk. It also provides two to three times the amount of the antioxidants lutein and zeaxanthin. Even though organic milk costs more (about an extra dollar a gallon), in this case, you really are getting the bang for your buck. One way to save money is to check organic company Web sites—Stonyfield Farm (stonyfield.com) and Organic Valley (organicvalley.coop) offer printable coupons online.

For more nutritional wisdom, insider secrets, and instant weight loss strategies, plus thousands of popular food comparisons, log on to **EATTHIS.COM.**

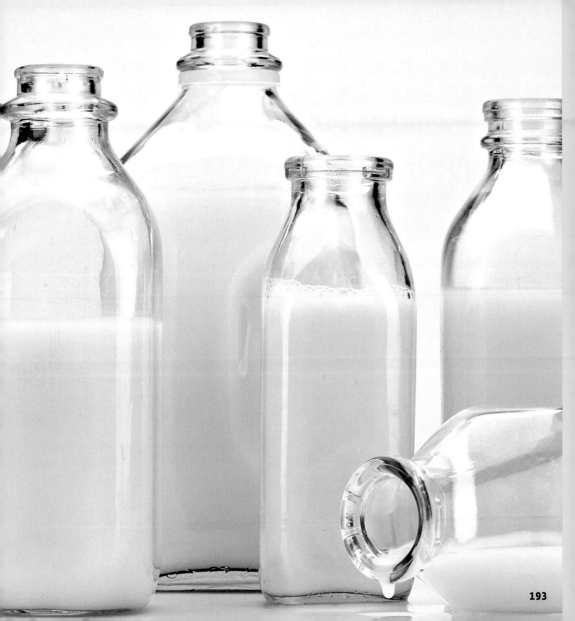

Making Sense of Milk

Untangling the mixed messages behind one of America's most misunderstood beverages

"Milk is a deadly poison," according to the Dairy Education Board. In fact, if you peruse this special interest group's Web site, notmilk.com, you'll find dozens of articles about the purported evils of this popular beverage. One claim, for example, is that milk from cows contains cancer-causing hormones and dairy industry dollars have kept that fact bottled up. All of which may leave you second-guessing your next sip.

And second-guessing is exactly what Americans have been doing lately. In the post-war days of 1945, the average American was consuming 45 gallons of milk a year. By 2001, with fears of saturated fat, high cholesterol, and high calories fomenting, per capita consumption was down to just 23 gallons.

Are we being fed mixed messages about milk? As is the case with most of the nutritional information we hear, the answer is yes. So to be sure it's safe, we've investigated all the anti-milk claims, sifting through the research while also turning a critical eye to pro-milk propaganda. After all, the only agenda we have is your health. The result: all your milk questions, answered.

Is milk really a fat-burning food?

Maybe. In a 6-month study, University of Tennessee researchers found that overweight people who downed three servings a day of calcium-rich dairy lost more belly fat than those who followed a similar diet minus two or more of the dairy servings. In addition, the researchers discovered that calcium supplements didn't work as well as milk. Why? They believe that while calcium may increase the rate at which your body burns fat, other active compounds in dairy (such as milk proteins) provide an additional fat-burning effect.

Does it build muscle?

Absolutely. In fact, milk is one of

the best muscle foods on the planet. You see, the protein in milk is about 80 percent casein and 20 percent whey. Both are high-quality proteins, but whey is known as a "fast protein" because it's quickly broken down into amino acids and absorbed into the bloodstream. That makes it a very good protein to consume after your workout. Casein, on the other hand, is digested more slowly. So it's ideal for providing your body with a steady supply of smaller amounts of protein for a longer period of time such as between meals or while you sleep.

Cows are given antibiotics. Doesn't that make their milk unhealthy?

No one really knows. Some scientists argue that milk from cows given antibiotics leads to antibiotic resistance in humans, making these types of drugs less effective when you take them for an infection. But this has never been proven.

It is true that hormones and antibiotics have never been part of a cow's natural diet, and they have been shown to have adverse effects on the animals. Canadian researchers, for example, discovered that cows given hormones are more likely to contract an udder infection called mastitis.

If you're uneasy, you can purchase antibiotic-free (and typically hormone-free, as well) milk from producers like Horizon and Organic Valley at most major supermarkets. The cows will certainly thank you.

Fat-free or whole?

It depends on your taste. While you've probably always been told to drink reduced-fat milk, the majority of scientific studies show that drinking whole milk actually improves cholesterol levels, just not as much as drinking fat-free does. One recent exception: Danish researchers found that men who consumed a diet rich in whole milk experienced a slight increase in LDL cholesterol (six points). However, it's worth noting that these men drank six 8-ounce glasses a day, an unusually high amount. Even so, their triglycerides—another marker of heart-disease risk—decreased by 22 percent.

The bottom line: Drinking two to three glasses of milk a day, whether it's fat-free, 2%, or whole, lowers the likelihood of both heart attack and stroke—a finding confirmed by British scientists.

From Cow to Carton
The magic behind milk's many manifestations

Back in the good old days, you always knew where your milk was coming from. If it wasn't from old Betsy out back, then the bottles were likely being delivered to your doorstep by a virtuous neighbor. But as the pastoral pleasantries of life as it once was have given way to the comforts and complexities of life as it now is, we've come to understand very little about where our food comes from—and that includes something as elemental as milk. Industrial farming practices have the whole process down to a firm science, one that takes billions of gallons of cream each year and efficiently divides them into milk's various permutations. Grab a glass; it's time for class:

1.
Cows are milked two to four times a day, and the raw milk they produce contains roughly 4 percent fat, 3 percent protein, 5 percent lactose sugar, and 87 percent water. The remaining fluid is filled with a variety of vitamins and minerals. 72 percent of the calcium in the American diet starts here, according to the USDA.

2.
After being transported to a processing plant, the raw milk is run through a centrifuge, a machine that spins like a dryer to separate the skim milk from the cream. ("Skimming" milk is an antiquated term. Maybe we should call it "spun milk," instead?)

3.
Now with two primary dairy components pulled apart, processors combine them back to form the gamut of dairy fluids. From skim milk and cream, we get the full dairy spectrum:

Cream
Even separated, cream is mostly water, but it does contain about 40 percent fat and a small dose of protein. Processors use small amounts of skim milk to thin out the fat and make the gamut of cream products. By the FDA's definition, light cream contains between 18 and 30 percent fat; whipping cream contains between 30 and 36 percent fat; and heavy cream contains no less than 36 percent fat. A cup of the heavy stuff has 414 calories.

6.
Finally the many faces of milk are packaged, shipped, and set out on display in your supermarket's dairy cooler.

5.
At this point most milk is fortified with vitamins A and D. The vitamin D aids in calcium absorption, protects your bones, and helps prevent cancer. The vitamin A improves skin, bolsters your immune system, and strengthens your eyes.

4.
The blended products are pasteurized, or heated momentarily to kill off potential pathogens, and then homogenized, which forces the erratic size fat globules through tiny holes so that they emerge consistently small and permanently suspended in the fluid.

Half and Half
Theoretically this is a 50-50 blend of whole milk and cream, but processors generally just blend skim milk and cream to achieve a fat concentration of 10.5 to 18 percent. A cup packs 315 calories, but a tablespoon in your coffee has just 20.

Whole Milk
It actually contains slightly less fat than it did in its raw form. FDA regulations mandate no less than 3.25 percent milk fat, so that's exactly what most processors use. Per 8 ounces, that works out to be 150 calories, 8 grams of fat, and 5 grams saturated.

Reduced-Fat Milk
Also known as 2% milk, because it contains 2% milk fat. Each serving has 8 grams of "complete" protein, which means it contains all the essential amino acids that your body can't make on its own.

Low-Fat Milk
The 1% compromise between skim and 2%. The difference between whole milk and low-fat milk is 40 calories. It might not sound like much, but that's 640 calories of savings per gallon.

Skim Milk
This is fat-free milk that has no cream added to it. Despite being the lowest in calories, this isn't always your best bet. Many of milk's nutrients—vitamins A and D, for instance—can't make it through your intestinal wall without the presence of fat.

Milk Alternatives

Feeling confined by the carton? Whether you're lactose intolerant or just monotony intolerant, there are plenty of other options out there beyond the regular moo juice, and most come with their own set of nutritional benefits. But before you expand your milk horizons, bone up on the array of alternatives—both popular and obscure—to ensure you stock your fridge with only the good stuff.

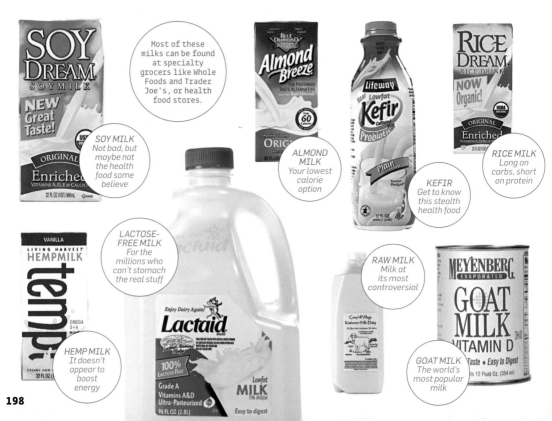

Most of these milks can be found at specialty grocers like Whole Foods and Trader Joe's, or health food stores.

SOY MILK
Not bad, but maybe not the health food some believe

ALMOND MILK
Your lowest calorie option

KEFIR
Get to know this stealth health food

RICE MILK
Long on carbs, short on protein

LACTOSE-FREE MILK
For the millions who can't stomach the real stuff

RAW MILK
Milk at its most controversial

HEMP MILK
It doesn't appear to boost energy

GOAT MILK
The world's most popular milk

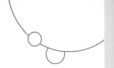

Raw Milk

Conventional milk goes through two processes before landing in the dairy cooler: pasteurization and homogenization. Pasteurization is the heating of milk to cook off dangerous pathogens, and homogenization is the process of forcing it through small holes to break down large fat globules and prevent the cream from rising to the top. But according to critics, both processes do more harm than good. Pasteurization, they claim, damages minerals such as calcium and iodine; and, according to a theory proposed in the '60s, homogenization can change the way our bodies absorb certain enzymes and increase our risk of heart disease. Truth is, most knocks against modernized milk are not yet backed by conclusive research. But talks about the dangers of raw milk tend to be similarly exaggerated. Unhomogenized milk doesn't pose any threats, but unpasteurized milk may; between 1998 and 2005,

the Centers for Disease Control and Prevention counted about a thousand reported illnesses resulting from raw milk consumption. Whether that amounts to a significant risk is your decision to make, but the FDA's stance is that the nutritional loss from pasteurization is somewhere between small and zilch. That's probably why pasteurization is endorsed by health-promoting organizations such as the American Medical Association and the American Academy of Pediatrics.

Per 8 fl oz (whole milk):
160 calories,
9 g fat (6 g saturated),
12 g sugars, 9 g protein

Soy Milk

Compared with most of the non-dairy milk alternatives, soy milk is the only one to boast a protein level similar to milk. That's probably why it's the only milk substitute to obtain the elevated status of a common household

grocery item. The concern with soy, however, is one that you won't notice by simply scanning the nutrition label. Two compounds buried inside the soybean, genistein and daidzein, function like mild estrogens in the body, which means they can disrupt your body's natural hormonal equilibrium. That can lead to reproductive problems in men, increased risk of breast cancer in women, and, according to a British study, double the risk of dementia and memory impairment in older people. Of course, other studies have shown beneficial and sometimes opposite effects, which incite inflamed debates from both sides of the health community. Bottom line: Until researchers figure it out, drink soy if you like, but keep consumption to a reasonable amount.

Per 8 fl oz: 132 calories,
4.5 g fat (0.5 g saturated),
10 g sugars, 8 g protein

Goat Milk

It might not be America's go-to milk, but in many of the world's less-developed countries, goat's milk is far more common than cow's. In fact, according to the American Dairy Goat Association, more people across the globe drink milk from goats than from any other animal. So how does it stack up against the milk you're used to? Unless you can find low-fat, goat milk can be high in calories, but it earns an advantage with slightly higher levels of calcium, phosphorus, potassium, and protein. And despite the lactose in goat milk, many people with dairy sensitivities still find it easier to digest. For those looking to avoid homogenized fats, goat milk provides one more advantage: Its fat globules are naturally small, so they don't require homogenization to prevent separation.

Per 8 fl oz: 168 calories,
10 g fat (7 g saturated),
11 g sugars, 9 g protein

Lactose-Free Milk

Lactose is the big sugar molecule that occurs naturally in milk, and in order to break it down into manageable pieces, most of our bodies produce an enzyme called lactase. For those who don't naturally produce the enzyme, drinking dairy milk can cause bloating, gas, diarrhea, and nausea. To get around this, food manufacturers treat milk with the lactase enzyme before they sell it. That way, the problematic lactose is broken down into two small, easy-to-digest sugar molecules called glucose and galactose. Unfortunately, that doesn't help people with true milk allergies; that's a problem with protein, not lactose. For those just needing a more digestable milk, look for lactose-free milk from companies like Lactaid and Organic Valley.

Per 8 fl oz (whole milk):
140 calories, 8 g fat
(3 g saturated), 14 g sugars,
10 g protein

Rice Milk

You can't expect the milk to be more nutritious than the grain that produced it, and that rule is best illustrated with rice milk. Rice consists of mostly starch, a carbohydrate that quickly breaks down to sugar in the body. Likewise, milk produced from rice is the most carbohydrate-rich of all the common nondairy milks. It's made by blending brown rice with water and straining out the solids, and it reaches the carton with a heavier load of calories than milk derived from seeds and nuts. One cup will run you about 120 calories, which is identical to 2% milk except that you've swapped out the protein for starch. Thankfully, manufacturers tend to fill out their cartons with heavy doses of calcium and B vitamins, thus saving their drinks from complete nutritional failure.

Per 8 fl oz: 120 calories,
2 g fat (0 g saturated),
25 g carbohydrates,
0.5 g protein

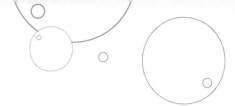

Kefir

This one's a bona fide stealth health food, creamier than milk and endowed with a heavier load of protein. That's because kefir is essentially drinkable yogurt. The process involves setting loose a cohort of yeast and bacteria to induce fermentation in the milk. The final product has low levels of lactose and high levels of probiotics, gut-friendly bacteria that promote healthy digestion. And what's more is that some animal and test-tube studies have suggested that kefir might be a formidable weapon against both cancer and heart disease. Calorically, kefir is on par with regular milk, but because it has a somewhat sour taste, it's often sweetened and blended with fruit. Be careful, though. Too much sugar and you could find yourself with a milk shake-like load of calories.

Per 8 fl oz (plain):
120 calories, 3 g fiber,
2 g fat (1.5 g saturated),
8 g sugars, 14 g protein

Hemp Milk

Much as with soy milk, hemp milk is made by the grinding of hemp seeds with water, sugar, and flavoring. The seed itself is loaded with healthy proteins, but by the time it's been processed, scarcely more than a couple grams will make it to your cup. But there's an upside. What this liquid lacks in protein it makes up for in healthy fats. A serving of hemp milk has about 7 grams of fat, and about 20 percent of those are omega-3s, the fatty acids that soften your arterial walls to improve your blood's ability to flow through your body. The downside is cost. Hemp milk is often priced at more than $5 a quart. Is it worth it? That's for you to decide.

Per 8 fl oz: 110 calories,
7 g fat (1 g saturated),
5 g sugars, 5 g protein

Almond Milk

Unsweetened almond milk carries about half as many calories as fat-free milk, which makes it the best dairy alternative for those trying to lose weight. Plus, to compete with the nutritional profile of cow's milk, brands such as Almond Breeze tend to lace their cartons with essential nutrients such as calcium and vitamins E and D. Of course, the low-calorie beverage can turn against you if it's loaded with sugar. Some of the flavored varieties (we're looking at you, chocolate) carry as much as 20 grams of sugar per serving, which will pack 80 extra calories into your 8-ounce glass. That's especially problematic considering almond milk carries scarcely any protein or fiber. If you must drink a sweetened beverage, aim for dairy or soy milk, both of which carry a load of protein to balance out the sugars.

Per 8 fl oz (sweetened):
70 calories, 2.5 g fat
(0 g saturated), 8 g sugars,
2 g protein

The Milk Shake Matrix
Master the art of the low-calorie drinkable dessert

With the exception of taking shots of melted butter or being hooked up to an IV of rendered bacon fat, there is no quicker way to put on pounds than to tussle with a restaurant-style milk shake. Think about it: ice cream, heavy cream or half and half, and a flood of different syrups and sweeteners, all whizzed together until you have a 1,000 calories or more than can be sucked down in 5 minutes flat.

But nobody is telling you to abandon the delicious genre entirely (well, at least we aren't). By making your next shake at home instead of grabbing it on the run, you'll not only save a few bucks, you'll save 500 calories or more per serving. Just follow these simple rules (or try one of our recipes) and you can have your shake and sip it too.

RULE #1
Build a better base

Most shakes start out with a high-fat, high-sugar base, either in the form of lackluster ice cream or the dreaded "dairy base," an amalgam of strange sweeteners, thickeners, and stabilizers. You'll save hundreds of calories simply by switching to frozen yogurt, or sticking with a reliable low-calorie ice cream brand, such as Breyers All Natural. More than that, you'll have a milk shake that is every bit like a shake was in the 1950s, back when they were made with just ice cream and milk. (Today, places such as Baskin-Robbins use 50 ingredients in some of their most diabolical concoctions.)

RULE #2
Master the mix

Milk shakes fail because most are made from 90 percent ice cream (or from an ice cream-like substance) concentrated in a drinkable form. Find other ways to stretch the shake and lighten the caloric load. Frozen fruit, 100 percent juice, ice, Greek yogurt: All will help you get more mileage out of your milk shake. Ultimately, you want no more than 1 cup of ice cream or frozen yogurt in your shake, and, to ensure the right consistency, no more than a half-cup of liquid. Also, it's essential to have a strong blender. A weak one will melt the ice cream and make for a watery milk shake.

RULE #3
Skip the sweeteners

Ice cream and frozen yogurt are sweet enough, so no need to grab for sugar or honey or anything else that will boost calories any higher than they already are. That also means go light on the cookies and cut out the candy bars. If there's one thing all of the worst shakes have in common, it's the inclusion of nougat-laced candy bars and cream-filled cookies. Want a cookies and cream shake? Skip the Oreos and use cookies and cream ice cream instead. Three Oreos will cost you 140 calories, but an upgrade from vanilla to cookies and cream ice cream should run you no more than 30.

RULE #4
Sneak in some nutrition

Just because it's dessert doesn't mean you can't conjure up some benefits in that frosty glass. The easiest way is to turn to the frozen banana: Not only does it add natural sweetness and a serving of fruit, but the frozen fruit also gives the milk shake a rich, creamy body and will help you cut back from the total ice cream allotment. The texture of frozen mango and peach chunks both pair beautifully with ice cream and fro-yo as well.

Even the smaller flavor add-ins can be relatively healthy. Peanut butter, fresh mint, and almonds all qualify.

The Grasshopper

2 cups Breyers All Natural Mint Chocolate Chip

1 cup fat-free milk

2 Thin Mint cookies, or other chocolate mint wafers

275 calories
4 g fat
41 g sugars

Almond Joy

2 cups Breyers All Natural Butter Almond ice cream

3 Tbsp coconut flakes

1 cup fat-free milk

390 calories
20 g fat
32 g sugars

Purple Cow

1 cup 100% grape juice

2 cups Breyers All Natural Vanilla

1 cup ice cubes

337 calories
6 g fat
54 g sugars

Strawberry Shortshake

1½ cups Breyers All Natural Strawberry Ice Cream

1 cup frozen strawberries

1 cup fat-free milk

6 vanilla wafers

Low-fat whipped cream for topping

315 calories
12 g fat
37 g sugars

Raspberry Mango Madness

2 cups frozen mango

2 cups raspberry sherbet or sorbet

1 cup fat-free milk

370 calories
0 g fat
75 g sugars

Peaches and Cream

2 cups low-fat vanilla frozen yogurt

2 cups frozen peaches

½ cup fat-free milk

340 calories
9 g fat
48 g sugars

All recipes yield 2 servings. Just throw the ingredients in a blender and puree.

BASKIN-ROBBINS

● The problem at Baskin-Robbins isn't limited to just a few egregious options; it's the virtual lack of anything remotely decent that earns them such dismal marks. The smallest size is a 16-ounce cup, which means even a small Light Shake can have close to 600 calories. All told, the average slurpable treat on the menu has 711 calories. The good news for ice cream lovers is that Baskin-Robbins's average scoop is well below the 200-calorie mark, making a small cup or cone a considerably healthier way to satisfy your dessert craving than nearly any of the dozens of deleterious drinks that pollute this menu.

Drink This

Ice Cream Float

(vanilla ice cream and root beer, small, 16 fl oz)

470 calories
20 g fat
(13 g saturated)
68 g sugars

Even with 140 calories more than the same float at A&W, this is one of the best options on Baskin's menu, which goes to show you just how dangerous drinks can be at the ice cream shop. Just be sure to watch your saturated fat intake for the rest of the day.

Other Picks

Wild Mango Fruit Blast
(small, 16 fl oz)
313 calories
1 g fat
(0 g saturated)
75 g sugars

Cappuccino Blast Made with Soft Serve
(small, 16 fl oz)
270 calories
6 g fat
(4 g saturated)
44 g sugars

Ice Cream Soda
(small, 16 fl oz)
480 calories
20 g fat
(13 g saturated,
0.5 g trans)
68 g sugars

Not That!

Vanilla Shake

(small, 16 fl oz)

670 calories
33 g fat
(21 g saturated,
1 g trans)
73 g sugars

Other Passes

Mango Fruit Cream

(small, 16 oz)
640 calories
18 g fat
(11 g saturated)
106 g sugars

Chocolate Shake
(with Premium Churned Light Milk Chocolate Ice Cream)

(small, 16 fl oz)
500 calories
16 g fat
(10 g saturated)
72 g sugars

Vanilla Shake
(made with Premium Churned Light Vanilla Ice Cream)

(medium, 24 fl oz)
820 calories
22 g fat
(14 g saturated)
128 g sugars

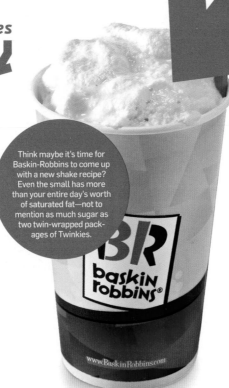

Think maybe it's time for Baskin-Robbins to come up with a new shake recipe? Even the small has more than your entire day's worth of saturated fat—not to mention as much sugar as two twin-wrapped packages of Twinkies.

www.BaskinRobbins.com

WEAPON OF MASS DESTRUCTION
Large Chocolate Chip Cookie Dough Shake
(32 fl oz)

1,690 calories
72 g fat (46 g saturated)
195 g sugars

Two years ago, Baskin-Robbins offered the worst beverage on the planet, a 2,600-calorie Oreo Shake. A hearty thanks to BR for finally removing that atrocity, but unfortunately, the legacy of waistline-expanding cookie-based shakes continues with this doughy disaster.

GUILTY PLEASURE

Premium Churned Light Aloha Brownie Ice Cream in a Cake Cone
(2.5 oz scoop)

175 calories
5 g fat (3 g saturated)
21 g sugars

Okay, it's not a beverage, but it's cold, it's creamy, and it will save you hundreds of calories over any drink on Baskin's menu. The Light Aloha Brownie is one of the few ice creams that the cold-cream mogul has dubbed a "BRight Choice."

BASKIN-ROBBINS *con't*

SUGAR SP↑KE

Large Mint Chocolate Chip Shake
(32 oz)

The Impact:

175 GRAMS!

Collectively, sugar and corn syrup show up six times on this shake's ingredient list, and between them they contribute 700 calories to the drink. That's in addition to the 670 calories of pure fat.

SIZE MATTERS!

CHOCOLATE CHIP COOKIE DOUGH SHAKE

LARGE

(32 fl oz)
1,690 calories

small

(16 fl oz)
750 calories

Total Savings: 940 CALORIES!

Drink This

Strawberry Citrus Fruit Blast

(small, 16 fl oz)

240 calories
0 g fat
58 g sugars

This is the lightest of the Fruit Blasts. It's also one of the best options on BR's drinks menu, offering what most other Baskin beverages can't: nutrients, in the form of real fruit purees that serve as the base of this drink.

Other Picks

Very Berry Strawberry Ice Cream
(2 scoops)
280 calories
14 g fat
(8 g saturated)
34 g sugars

Freeze
(with orange sherbet)
(small, 16 fl oz)
370 calories
4 g fat
(2.5 g saturated)
81 g sugars

Oreo Cookies 'n Cream Ice Cream
(2 scoops, in a Cake Cone)
365 calories
18 g fat
(10 g saturated)
34 g sugars

440 calories
1.5 g fat
(0 g saturated)
101 g sugars

Not That!

Mango Fruit Blast Smoothie

(small, 16 fl oz)

Other Passes

Strawberry Shake

(small, 16 fl oz)

560 calories
23 g fat
(15 g saturated,
1 g trans)
73 g sugars

Raspberry Chip Shake

(medium, 24 fl oz)

760 calories
21 g fat
(14 g saturated)
117 g sugars

Oreo 'N Cookies Cappuccino Blast

(medium, 24 fl oz)

740 calories
31 g fat
(21 g saturated)
73 g sugars

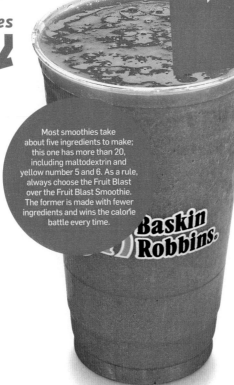

Most smoothies take about five ingredients to make; this one has more than 20, including maltodextrin and yellow number 5 and 6. As a rule, always choose the Fruit Blast over the Fruit Blast Smoothie. The former is made with fewer ingredients and wins the calorie battle every time.

Baskin Robbins.

BEVERAGE MYTH

Smoothies are as healthy as real fruit.

Most commercially prepared smoothies suffer two punishing flaws: an abundance of added sugar and a lack of the fiber found in whole fruit. That's how a Mango Blast Smoothie at Baskin-Robbins squeezes in twice as much sugar—and only a third as much fiber—as a same-size cup of fresh sliced mango.

For 900 calories, you can have

ALL THIS

Two Scoops of Chocolate Chip Ice Cream in a Sugar Cone, One Scoop of Strawberry Sorbet, One Mango Fruit Blast Bar, and a Reese's Peanut Butter Sundae Cup

 OR

THAT

A Medium Chocolate Chip Shake (19 fl oz)

COLD STONE CREAMERY

● On one side of the menu they have some of the worst shakes in the country, but on the other they have a full line of smoothies that rivals the fruity purees put out by big-smoothie operators Jamba Juice and Smoothie King. Still, outside of that there's plenty of room for caloric catastrophe. The coffee drinks are loaded with sugar, and the "sinless" shakes— although a massive step ahead of the regular line—are slightly more nefarious than the name suggests.

Drink This

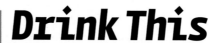

Iced Milk Caramel Latte

with whipped cream (Like It size, 16 oz)

360 calories
17 g fat
(13 g saturated)
37 g sugars

Other Picks

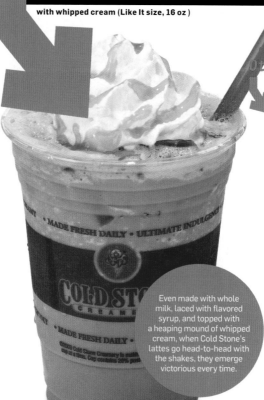

Even made with whole milk, laced with flavored syrup, and topped with a heaping mound of whipped cream, when Cold Stone's lattes go head-to-head with the shakes, they emerge victorious every time.

Blueberry Pineapple Smoothie
(Love It size, 20 oz)
360 calories
5 g fat
(3.5 g saturated)
53 g sugars

Strawberry Bananza Smoothie
(Gotta Have It, 24 oz)
240 calories
2 g fat
(0 g saturated)
37 g sugars

Sinless Oh Fudge Shake
(Like It size, 16 oz)
490 calories
2 g fat
(2 g saturated)
44 g sugars

1,742

The number of calories in the average Gotta Have It-size shake

Not That!

Lotta Caramel Latte Shake

(Like It size, 16 oz)

1,320 calories
62 g fat
(39 g saturated)
134 g sugars

Other Passes

Mango Pineapple Smoothie

(Love It size, 20 oz)

510 calories
5 g fat
(3.5 g saturated)
83 g sugars

Banana Strawberry Smoothie

(Gotta Have It size, 24 oz)

450 calories
6 g fat
(3.5 g saturated)
64 g sugars

Sinless Cake n Shake

(Like It size, 16 oz)

670 calories
7 g fat
(2 g saturated)
57 g sugars

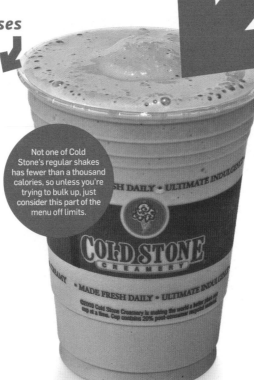

Not one of Cold Stone's regular shakes has fewer than a thousand calories, so unless you're trying to bulk up, just consider this part of the menu off limits.

For 1,390 calories, you can have

ALL THIS

A Love It Vanilla Bean Ice Cream with Chocolate Shavings, Blueberries, and Hot Fudge; a Gotta Have It Raspberry Sorbet; and a Like It Vanilla Crème Latte

OR

THAT

A Love It Very Vanilla Shake
(20 oz)

DAIRY QUEEN

● DQ serves up some of the most bloated beverages in the nation. Its average drink weighs in at a staggering 649 calories, and that's not even factoring in the horrendous line of Blizzards. The long line of shakes and MooLattes lack a low-fat counterpart to even them out. For an occasional treat, DQ won't kill you, but never use one of these ice-cream beverages to wash down a burger and fries.

Drink This

Banana Shake

(small, 14 fl oz)

450 calories
14 g fat
(9 g saturated,
0.5 g trans)
55 g sugars

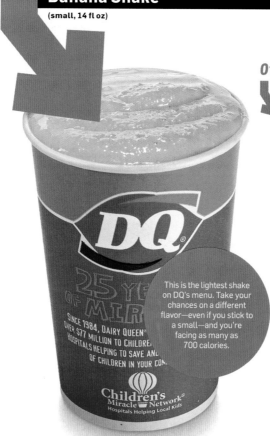

This is the lightest shake on DQ's menu. Take your chances on a different flavor—even if you stick to a small—and you're facing as many as 700 calories.

Other Picks

Chocolate Sundae (small) and Coffee
(12 fl oz)
285 calories
7 g fat
(4.5 g saturated)
41 g sugars

Arctic Rush
(medium, 21 fl oz)
310 calories
0 g fat
63 g sugars

Arctic Rush
(small, 16 oz)
240 calories
0 g fat
48 g sugars

185

The number of times you'd have to ice skate the perimeter of an NHL ice rink to burn the 830 calories in a large Mocha MooLatte

700 calories
23 g fat
(16 g saturated,
1 g trans)
85 g sugars

Not That!
Hot Fudge Malt Shake
(small, 15.1 fl oz)

Other Passes

Mocha Moo Latte
(16 fl oz)
590 calories
23 g fat
(15 saturated,
0.5 g trans)
72 g sugars

Minute Maid Orange Float
(medium, 22.5 fl oz)
500 calories
9 g fat
(6 g saturated,
0.5 g trans)
71 g sugars

Arctic Rush Freeze
(small, 14 oz)
440 calories
11 g fat
(8 g saturated,
0.5 g trans)
61 g sugars

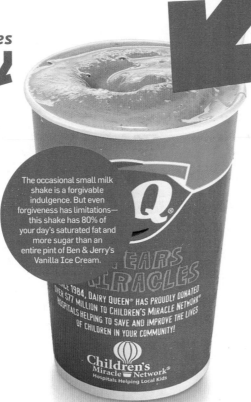

The occasional small milk shake is a forgivable indulgence. But even forgiveness has limitations—this shake has 80% of your day's saturated fat and more sugar than an entire pint of Ben & Jerry's Vanilla Ice Cream.

SINCE 1984, DAIRY QUEEN® HAS PROUDLY DONATED OVER $77 MILLION TO CHILDREN'S MIRACLE NETWORK® HOSPITALS HELPING TO SAVE AND IMPROVE THE LIVES OF CHILDREN IN YOUR COMMUNITY!

Children's Miracle Network®
Hospitals Helping Local Kids

SUGAR SPIKE
Large Pineapple Malt
The Impact:
153 GRAMS!
This cup carries more sugar than an entire carton of Edy's Slow Churned French Vanilla Ice Cream. Oh, and it has 1,130 calories and a full day's saturated fat. This is what happens when fruit gets into the wrong hands.

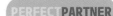

PERFECT PARTNER

Original Hamburger
350 calories
14 g fat
(7 g saturated)
680 mg sodium

The problem is the burger-and-shake shop's "eats" menu is as riddled with fat as the "treats" menu is with sugar. Stick to regular-size entrées and skip the sides. You won't turn out a truly nutritious meal, but you will fight off the pudgy guilt of eater's remorse.

Drink This

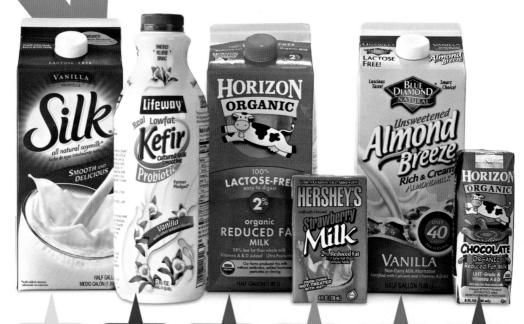

Silk Vanilla
(8 fl oz)

100 calories
3.5 g fat
(0.5 g
saturated)
7 g sugars

Just goes to show
you that often
times choosing
a flavor is as
important as
picking a brand.

Lifeway
Lowfat Kefir
Vanilla (8 fl oz)

160 calories
2 g fat
(1.5 g
saturated)
21 g sugars

Kefir is a creamy,
yogurt-like drink
loaded with protein,
fiber, and gut-
friendly bacteria.

Horizon
Organic
Lactose-Free
2% Milk (8 fl oz)

120 calories
5 g fat
(3 g saturated)
12 g sugars

About 30 million
Americans have
trouble processing
lactose. This is the
best solution.

Hershey's
2% Milk
Strawberry
(8 fl oz box)

170 calories
5 g fat
(3 g saturated)
25 g sugars

Even though this
one wins out,
strawberry milk is
more a dessert
than a daily drink.

Blue Diamond
Almond
Breeze
Vanilla (8 fl oz)

40 calories
3 g fat
(0 g saturated)
0 g sugars

Fortified with half
your daily vitamin
E, which helps
keep your skin
looking young.

Horizon
Chocolate
Organic
Reduced Fat
Milk (8 fl oz box)

180 calories
5 g fat
(3 g saturated)
27 g sugars

Horizon makes
the best on-the-
go milks on
the market.

Not That!

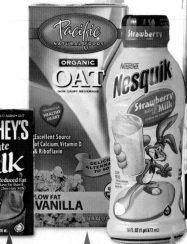

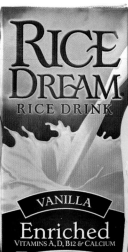

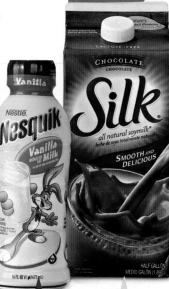

Hershey's Chocolate 2% Milk
(8 fl oz box)

200 calories
5 g fat
(3 g saturated)
29 g sugars

Horizon delivers the same stuff for fewer calories and no hormones or antibiotics.

Pacific Foods Low-Fat Vanilla Oat Milk (8 fl oz)

130 calories
2.5 g fat
(0 g saturated)
20 g sugars

Thank the high sugar load for bumping this one into the "That" category.

Nesquik Reduced Fat Milk Strawberry
(8 fl oz)

200 calories
5 g fat
(3 g saturated)
30 g sugars

Hershey's offers a nearly identical product with 30 fewer calories.

Rice Dream Enriched Vanilla
(8 fl oz)

130 calories
2.5 g fat
(0 g saturated)
12 g sugars

Rice milk is relatively high in calories and low in nutrients. Not a good sub for milk.

Nesquik Reduced Fat Vanilla Milk
(8 fl oz)

190 calories
5 g fat
(3 g saturated)
29 g sugars

Switch to Kefir and you'll get a creamier treat with a better array of nutrients.

Silk Chocolate
(8 fl oz)

140 calories
3 g fat
(0.5 g saturated)
19 g sugars

Don't make the mistake of thinking that soy milk is a stealth health food.

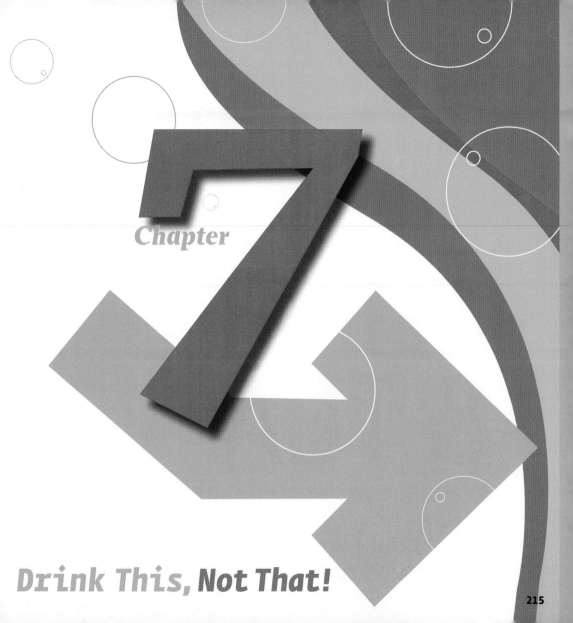

Drink This, Not That!

COFFEE & TEA

What's more comforting than a warm mug of fresh coffee? What could be more peaceful than a nice, quiet cup of tea?

CHAPTER 7

This is what you drink first thing in the morning as you read the paper, or over scones with your aging great-aunt, or while you're meeting up for business conversation with colleagues. Coffee or tea is what you suggest to someone you're interested in, when you don't want to tip them off to the fact that you're interested. They're perfect because they're perfectly innocent.

But the fact is, tea and coffee have nothing on beer and whiskey when it comes to causing chaos, arousing passions, and even inciting bloodshed. Coffee, after all, has been put on trial in Mecca, was first introduced into Europe by smugglers, and is banned to this day by the Mormon faith. Coffeehouses are where the beatniks dreamed up angry American culture and the grunge rockers dreamed up angry American music. (And, to be honest, I'm pretty damn ornery before I get my morning coffee, too, so watch out, pal.) Tea, on the other hand, was a main driver behind the opium wars, became a symbol of the patriots' rebellion against the British, and to

this day serves as the rallying cry of really, really angry Americans who want to get rid of most of Congress. In fact, no two beverages have started so many military conflicts—or changed the face of the globe nearly as much.

The funny thing is, while beer and whisky may have the reputation as troublemakers (no band of gunslingers ever sidled up to a bar and demanded chai), tea and coffee are the drinks that are really worth fighting over. Why? Because both seem to have magical properties that help us diminish hunger. (Cool slice of trivia to whip out next time you're flirting with a barista: Some lexicographers believe the word "coffee" comes from the Arabic qahiya, which means "to have no appetite," because the brew has long been known to quell hunger.)

But they do more than that: They actually cause our bodies to burn calories faster! A study published in the journal *Physiology and Behavior* found that the average metabolic rate of people who drank caffeinated coffee was 16 percent higher than those who drank decaf. Other studies have found that caffeinated coffee can rev your metabolism to burn as many as 174 additional calories a day. (That's the equivalent of burning off a pound and a half of flab every 20 days!)

And tea may be an even more potent weapon against obesity. Canadian researchers found that men who drink more than 2 cups of tea a day have slimmer waistlines than those who drink none. (Artificial sweetener alert: In the same study, men who added sugar to their tea had waist measurements 1 inch smaller than the general population; but men who added artificial sweeteners had waistlines

Breaking Down the Buzz

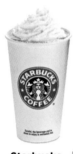 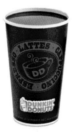 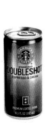 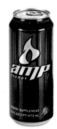 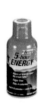 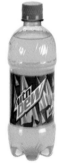

Starbucks Caffè Mocha (grande, 16 fl oz)	**Dunkin' Donuts Black Coffee** (medium, 14 fl oz)	**Starbucks DoubleShot Coffee Drink** (1 can, 8 fl oz)**	**AMP Energy** (1 can, 16 fl oz)	**5-Hour Energy** (1 shot, 2 fl oz)	**Mountain Dew** (1 bottle, 20 fl oz)
Caffeine: 175 mg	Caffeine: 164 mg	Caffeine: 160 mg	Caffeine: 143 mg	Caffeine: 135 mg	Caffeine: 91 mg
Sugars: 33 g	Sugars: 0 g	Sugars: 21 g	Sugars: 58 g	Sugars: not given	Sugars: 77 g
Calories: 330	Calories: 10	Calories: 170	Calories: 220	Calories: 4	Calories: 290

**Note that the DoubleShot Energy + Coffee of the same size has about 80 fewer milligrams of caffeine*

that were 2 inches bigger!) One Japanese study found that a cup of brewed tea can raise your metabolism by 12 percent; in another study, men given green tea extract showed a 4 percent boost in total energy expenditure. And studies also show that black tea may help control surges in blood sugar, effectively lowering your risk of diabetes.

If this all sounds like carte blanche to indulge in coffee and tea no matter where you find it, tap the brakes a few times before you head out the door. Coffee and tea may be miracles of nature, but like many of the world's great wonders (such as the American economy, Michael Jackson, or cheese

Calculating the caffeine content in America's most popular beverages

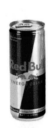 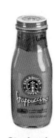 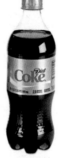 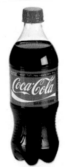 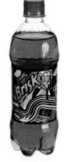 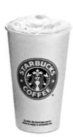

Red Bull	**Starbucks**	**Diet Coke**	**Coca-Cola**	**Lipton Brisk**	**Starbucks**
(1 can, 8.4 fl oz)	**Frappuccino**	(1 bottle, 20 fl oz)	**Classic**	**Lemon**	**Decaf Latte**
Caffeine:	**Coffee Drink**	**Caffeine:**	(1 bottle, 20 fl oz)	**Iced Tea**	(grande, 16 fl oz)
80 mg	(1 bottle,	**76.6 mg**	**Caffeine:**	(1 bottle, 20 fl oz)	**Caffeine:**
Sugars: 27 g	8 fl oz)**	Sugars: 0 g	**56.7 mg**	**Caffeine:**	**13 mg**
Calories: 110	**Caffeine:**	Calories: 0	Sugars: 65 g	**14 mg**	Sugars: 17 g
	76 mg		Calories: 233	Sugars: 55 g	Calories: 190
	Sugars: 27 g			Calories: 210	
	Calories: 170				

**This drink also available in 9.5 fl oz and 13.7 fl oz bottles; caffeine in the 13.7 fl oz bottle is 130 mg

pizza), somebody looking to make a fast buck (international bankers, plastic surgeons, whoever invented "stuffed crust") will come up with a way to mess everything up by "improving" them. And so it's been with coffee and tea. Today, your average convenience store is brimming with coffee and tea drinks, but those beverages don't have the amazing weight-loss qualities that the originals had. Most iced teas, iced coffees, and fancy high-concept concoctions from the local coffeehouse come loaded with sugar, fat, and chemicals—ingredients that will slow your metabolism and bolster weight gain. A Starbucks venti Caramel Frappuccino Blended Coffee, for example, will take what should be a 5-calorie coffee drink and turn it into a 500-calorie meal. (The good news: You'll burn off half of those calories just trying to pronounce this monster.)

So how do you get the magical weight-loss properties of tea and coffee without the magical weight-gain properties that food and beverage purveyors want to saddle us with? By knowing which drinks are still good for your waistline, and which have been turned into stealth health-busters. Fortunately, we've done the homework. The cheat sheet is right in your hands!

Know Your Joe

Coffee is the world's most popular fix. And yet it's hard to know what to make of the mixed messages about its effects on our health. We want to set the record straight: Coffee, down to its deep, dark, caffeine-filled soul, is good for you. And that's good, because four out of five American adults drink the heady brew.

"Coffee is one of the most heavily researched products in the world today," says Roger Cook, director of the Coffee Science Information Center. "And the vast majority of this research clearly shows that drinking coffee can be quite beneficial to your health." Of course he'd say that. But the research backs it up. That morning cup can help decrease your risk of Parkinson's disease, Alzheimer's disease, and type 2 diabetes. But there's a difference between a healthy love and a dubious addiction. Pour yourself a second cup and read on.

The Bean

Out of the nearly 100 varieties of coffee beans, only two make their way to the cup. Arabica, known for its deep, complex flavor, accounts for about 75 percent of the beans sold throughout the world. Robusta, a cheaper bean usually considered a filler, is often found lurking in the canisters you buy in the supermarket.

- *Robusta beans are found in standard supermarket brands.*
- *Most small-batch, specialty roasters use arabica beans.*
- *Instant coffee? Don't go there.*

The Roast

"The darker the roast, the fewer characteristics of the bean you taste," says Kenneth Davids, a cofounder of CoffeeReview.com. Most single-origin coffees, such as Colombian, Sumatra, and other coffees named after countries, are lightly roasted to preserve the beans' natural flavor. Blends are typically roasted for a desired flavor. The three main categories:

Medium: *These coffees are roasted for 9 to 11 minutes, like most grocery-store varieties. Also called breakfast roast.*

Dark: *In this common European method, batches are roasted for 12 to 13 minutes until the oils reach the surface of the beans. Also called French roast.*

Extra Dark: *Roasted for at least 14 minutes, these oily beans taste so smoky that it's tough to identify where they were grown. You drink it for the deep roast, not the nuance of the bean. Also called Italian or Espresso roast.*

Beware of flavored beans—these are usually cheap robusta beans roasted to oblivion and flavored artificially. If you need a hazelnut or vanilla fix, buy a bottle of flavored oil and mix a teaspoon into the good stuff.

The Region

All good coffee is grown between the Tropic of Cancer and the Tropic of Capricorn, where the climate is ideal for producing rich, full-flavored beans. Each of the three major coffee-growing regions produces a distinct flavor. Known for their lighter coffees, the Americas produce more joe than any other region. "Latin American coffee's crisp, bright acidity comes as a direct result of its climate and the volcanic soils the beans grow in," says Andy Fouché, a certified coffee specialist, formerly with Starbucks Coffee. Africa/Arabia, the region where coffee was born 1,200 years ago, produces a smoother, less acidic cup than the Americas. The Asia/Pacific region produces the boldest of coffees, often with a heavy, earthy taste.

The Brew

Even the most carefully roasted beans can be ruined by sloppy brewing. Start by buying your coffee fresh in small batches every 2 weeks. Skip the preground stuff and buy your beans whole instead; grinding them just before you brew will make the best cup. For a standard drip machine, use filtered water and about 2 tablespoons of ground beans for every 6 ounces of brewed coffee. Pack the grounds tightly into the filter, eliminating air between the grounds, for a richer brew. When it comes to storing your beans, keep them out of the freezer—it destroys the essential oils that make coffee delicious. Keep beans in your cupboard in an airtight container.

The Buzz

"Seventy percent of people's daily caffeine consumption comes from coffee," says Joe Vinson, PhD, a professor of chemistry at the University of Scranton, in Pennsylvania. Caffeine content is determined by the type of bean and the way the beans are roasted and prepared. Arabica beans have about 1 percent caffeine, while robusta beans have twice that (meaning that crappy cup from the gas station may have double the dosage). Roasting reduces the caffeine content—so stronger-tasting coffee doesn't necessarily mean more caffeine. Here's an eye-opener: According to Illy Coffee, a shot of its espresso has 35 percent less caffeine than the company's brewed coffee.

The Benefits

Pure, black coffee is one of the world's most potent elixirs. "Generally, drinking 1 to 3 cups a day will increase your overall health," says Vinson, who recently discovered that coffee is the number one source of antioxidants in the American diet. These antioxidants have been shown to possibly prevent certain types of cancer, including colorectal, and reduce the risk of developing alcoholic cirrhosis by 22 percent. Moreover, the neurological impact of caffeine has been shown to slow the aging process and enhance short-term-memory performance. But keep your coffee intake to four 8-ounce cups a day; after that, the benefits are outweighed by an increased risk of hypertension and cardiovascular disease.

The Life of a Bean

From tree to cup to brain

Planting

After planting, coffee trees take about 2 years to develop fragrant, white flowers. As the flowers mature, a fruit, usually called a coffee cherry, is formed. The cherry matures in anywhere from 6 to 11 months and is then harvested and processed.

Processing

There are three main ways coffee cherries are processed: wet, dry, and semidry. In wet processing, the fruit of the cherry is washed away, leaving the pit, a.k.a. the coffee bean. Dry-processed cherries are placed in the sun until the fruit is dried off the bean, which produces a sweeter flavor. Semidry is a combination of the two, and it's gaining popularity because it combines the sweet flavor of dry processing with some of the ease of wet processing.

Roasting

Roasting can be done anywhere from a factory to your home oven. Bringing out the richness in a raw bean without destroying its inherent flavor is a delicate art. "A medium roast of a good coffee is like a nice table wine—really bright with that pleasant acidity," says Kenneth Davids, a cofounder of CoffeeReview.com. But an over-roasted bean can be like bad box wine, lacking any subtlety or balance.

Preparing

Good coffee is about proper flavor extraction from the bean, and each brewing method demands a different grind. French presses and percolators use the coarsest grind (about 5 to 10 seconds in your grinder); automatic-drip machines need a medium grind (10 to 15 seconds); and espresso machines require the finest grind (25 seconds).

Metabolizing

Within about 15 minutes of your first sip, the caffeine starts the release of dopamine in your brain's prefrontal cortex. This effect, which increases wakefulness and mental focus, among other things, peaks in about 30 minutes.

Countertop Coffee Bar

1 BEST WAY TO GET YOUR GRIND ON

Capresso Black Burr Grinder

$50, capresso.com

Talk to serious coffee guys and they all say the same thing: The easiest way to mess up a cup of coffee or an espresso is to use a standard metal blade grinder. "To make great coffee, you need the grounds to all be about the same size," says Billy Wilson, owner of Barista in Portland, Oregon. "A whirly blade grinder indiscriminately grinds the coffee into all shapes and sizes. But a burr grinder won't release the grounds until they're uniform." Capresso has been in the business of burr grinding for many years and still makes some of the most reliable, affordable products.

2 BEST ESPRESSO ON A SHOESTRING

Bialetti Moka Express 3-Cup Espresso Maker

$25, bialettishop.com

While baristas across the Boot grapple with $10,000 machines, most Italians make their espresso on the stovetop, and no device is more ubiquitous than this

simple Moka maker. Just pack the bottom with quality grounds, turn on the stove, and 5 minutes later, you'll have a thick, rich cup of caffeinated goodness.

3 BEST ESPRESSO MACHINE FOR THE OCCASIONAL LATTE

Dé Longhi EC 155

$100, delonghiusa.com

It won't whisk you back to that first shot you took in a Roman café, but for the money, we haven't found a better machine capable of producing a strong shot of espresso with a nice cap of crema.

Brew This: Illy Easy Serving Espresso Pods ($27 for 36 pods, illyusa. com). You'll have a great shot with no cleanup. Don't dig the pods? The Dé Longhi takes freshly ground espresso, too.

4 BEST WAY TO MAKE YOUR FAVORITE COFFEE EVERY MORNING

Bunn NHBX-B Contemporary 10-Cup Home Coffee Brewer

$90, amazon.com

Bunn has long supplied the restaurant industry with its coffee makers, but this machine pumps out

10 cups of exceptional coffee in 3 minutes flat for the discerning (and time-pressed) home brewer. Plus, its stainless steel tank keeps water hot for tea and other uses.

Brew This: Counter Culture La Golondrina ($11.75 per 12-ounce bag, counterculturecoffee. com). This North Carolina-based coffee roaster sources its beans directly from small artisanal farmers from around the world. La Golondrina, from a farm in Columbia, makes a beautifully balanced cup of coffee with notes of chocolate and cherry. Or, if you pledge allegiance to grocery-store grounds, use Chock Full o'Nuts ($4 for 13 ounces), the deepest-bodied bean we found in the aisles.

5 MACHINE MOST LIKELY TO REPLACE YOUR STARBUCKS HABIT

Dé Longhi ESAM3300 Magnifica Super-Automatic Espresso

$800, amazon.com

Program your favorite drinks, then simply press a button and kick back while the machine grinds and processes your beans into thick, rich, soul-

soothing espresso shots, Americanos, and even normal (but excellent) cups of coffee. It's expensive, yes, but if you're the type to drop $5 a day at the local coffee shop, this baby would be a wise investment.

Brew This: Intelligentsia's Black Cat Espresso Blend ($11 per pound, intelligentsiacoffee.com). The heavy-bodied bean with a rich caramel finish came out flawlessly from the Pro Line every time.

6 BEST WAY TO WHIP IT

BonJour Primo Latte Frother

$20, bonjourproducts.com

Even the frothers on the most expensive home espresso machines are often disappointing. We usually ignore them entirely when we're in the mood for a cappuccino and instead turn to this little magic wand. It weighs less than a pound but can whip your milk into a frothy, feathery frenzy in a matter of seconds. Just remember, cold skim milk is best for frothing. Froth for 20 to 30 seconds in a microwave-safe glass, then heat for 30 seconds for hot milk and stable foam.

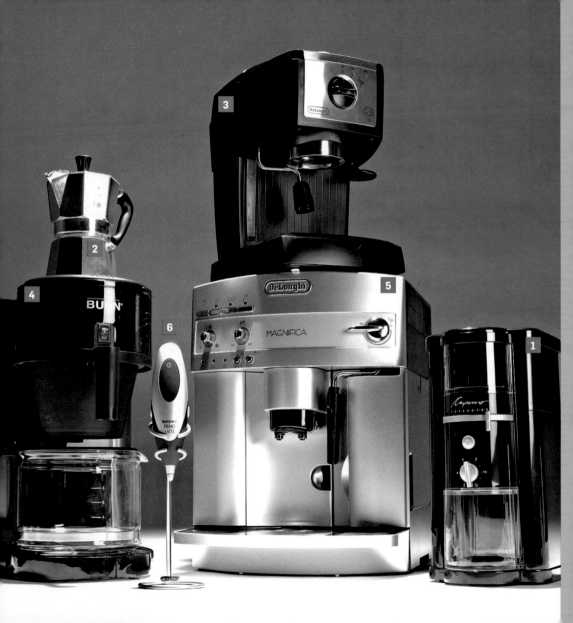

What the Beans Really Mean

Decode the industry jargon and make sure you're getting your money's worth

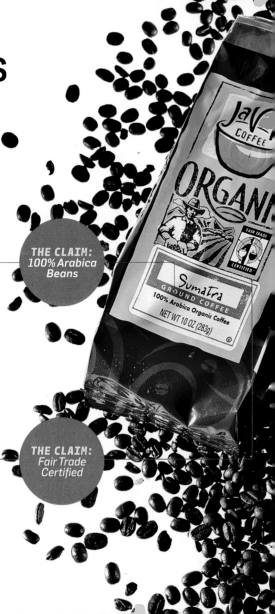

THE CLAIM:
100% Arabica Beans

THE TRUTH:

Coffee beans come in two main varieties: arabica and robusta. Of the two, arabica beans deliver the most complex flavors, but because they're more difficult to grow—i.e., more expensive—commercial roasters such as Folgers often fill out their blends with cheap robusta beans. That makes for a cup with big body but low acid, which means it's heavy in the mouth but not particularly interesting to the tongue. Small-scale craft roasters don't generally bother putting this information on the bag, but that's fine considering most of them wouldn't dare to pollute their coffee with robustas. But when you're shopping the commercial blends in the super-market, you should seek this claim.

THE CLAIM:
Fair Trade Certified

THE TRUTH:

Much of the world's coffee is grown in impoverished countries where farmers struggle to feed their families, and fair trade certification is the cooperative effort to change this. Right now that means US importers pay farmers no less than $1.35 per pound of conventional coffee and $1.51 per pound of organic. That would have been huge in 2001 when the year's average was $.46 per pound, but today the average farmer sells at more than $1.20, according to the International Coffee Organization. Furthermore, some journalists have uncovered instances where fair trade farmers were making less than the minimum wage set by their government, and some economists argue that the artificial price floor creates a surplus for fair trade coffee that ultimately drives down the price of noncertified beans. That being said, most fair trade coffee is also organic, and many struggling farmers have improved their lives by working with fair trade organizations.

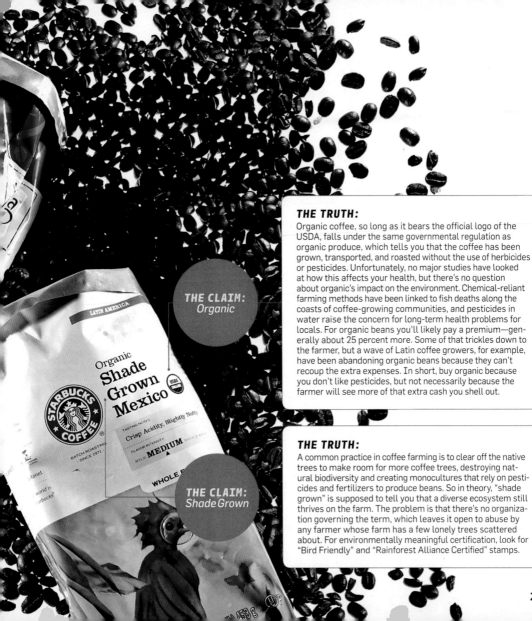

THE CLAIM:
Organic

THE TRUTH:
Organic coffee, so long as it bears the official logo of the USDA, falls under the same governmental regulation as organic produce, which tells you that the coffee has been grown, transported, and roasted without the use of herbicides or pesticides. Unfortunately, no major studies have looked at how this affects your health, but there's no question about organic's impact on the environment. Chemical-reliant farming methods have been linked to fish deaths along the coasts of coffee-growing communities, and pesticides in water raise the concern for long-term health problems for locals. For organic beans you'll likely pay a premium—generally about 25 percent more. Some of that trickles down to the farmer, but a wave of Latin coffee growers, for example, have been abandoning organic beans because they can't recoup the extra expenses. In short, buy organic because you don't like pesticides, but not necessarily because the farmer will see more of that extra cash you shell out.

THE CLAIM:
Shade Grown

THE TRUTH:
A common practice in coffee farming is to clear off the native trees to make room for more coffee trees, destroying natural biodiversity and creating monocultures that rely on pesticides and fertilizers to produce beans. So in theory, "shade grown" is supposed to tell you that a diverse ecosystem still thrives on the farm. The problem is that there's no organization governing the term, which leaves it open to abuse by any farmer whose farm has a few lonely trees scattered about. For environmentally meaningful certification, look for "Bird Friendly" and "Rainforest Alliance Certified" stamps.

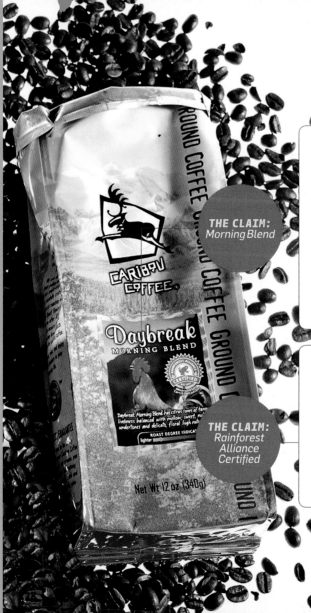

THE CLAIM:
Morning Blend

THE CLAIM:
Rainforest Alliance Certified

THE TRUTH:

A blend is simply a mix of beans from at least two different regions, and a "morning blend" is whatever that particular roaster thought you might enjoy at the start of the day. In contrast with blends are the single-origin coffees, which are identified simply by their place of origin: Brazil, Columbia, Ethiopia, or whatever the case may be. Presumably the goal with blending is to create a better-tasting cup, but often that's not the case. Some roasters blend to bury the mistakes of flawed beans, and many connoisseurs find the pure flavors of single-origin coffee more satisfying than blends. And get this: When *Consumer Reports* recently rated 37 popular blends from places such as Starbucks, Peets, Caribou, and Green Mountain Coffee Roasters, not one of them was considered good enough to earn the top scores of "excellent" or "very good."

THE TRUTH:

Rainforest Alliance Certified must meet a strict set of requirements that promote sustainable resource management and the preservation of healthy ecosystems. That means farms must be partially covered by native trees, farmers must make living wages, and farming methods must have a minimal impact on the natural environment. The only designation more meaningful than the Rainforest Alliance Certification is the Bird Friendly stamp. Bird Friendly coffees have similarly strict eco standards, but they require the farm to also be certified organic, whereas the Rainforest Alliance allows the use of some chemicals.

How to make perfect iced coffee

Coffee, in its brain-preserving, diabetes-defending, cancer-fighting glory, may be one of the world's most enjoyable superfoods. But as the mercury climbs, the quality of your caffeine fix plummets. That's because most coffee shops charge extra for iced coffee, only to melt a feeble cup of cubes with piping-hot java. (Yeah, that's why your iced coffee at Starbucks tastes so weak.) Skip the diluted version and cold-brew a batch at home.

Combine ⅔ cup of coffee grounds and 3 cups of cold water in a glass jar or French press, stir, and let the brew sit overnight. In the morning, pour it through a sieve (or lower the French press plunger) to strain out the grounds. Combine this concentrate with an equal amount of cold water. As for the cubes? Make them with the concentrate: As they melt, your joe gets better.

Of course, the effort is wasted if you don't start with good beans. Luckily, the artisan coffee movement is fully percolating in the US. Among our favorite coffees right now are the Panama Esmeralda Especial from Stumptown Coffee Roasters (stumptowncoffee.com) and the Finca Santuario from Intelligentsia Coffee (intelligentsiacoffee.com).

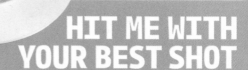

HIT ME WITH YOUR BEST SHOT

"Espresso is all about the crema," says Matt Riddle, a designer for Intelligentsia Coffee and the 2006 winner of the United States Barista Championship. "Think of a Guinness when it's poured; that's how the shot should look—a nice dark body, but with a reddish brown top." Achieve crema perfection and espresso ecstasy in five steps:

1 **The bean:** Find the "Roasted On" or "Best Before" date and make sure the coffee's less than 2 weeks out of the roaster. "Coffee is a food; it can spoil like anything else in your cupboard," says Riddle.

2 **The grind:**** Use a burr grinder to make sure the beans are ground evenly. Setting the grinder on the finest setting should make the grinds about the size of table salt.

3 **The tamp:** Fill your basket until there's a quarter inch of room at the top. Now press down with your tamper, using about 30 pounds of pressure. "Use a normal bathroom scale to see how much force you need," says Riddle. Then tightly place the basket in the machine.

4 **The water:** Make sure the temperature is between 198°F and 204°F and the pressure is around 8 or 9 bars. The 2-ounce shot should take between 20 and 30 seconds to pour.

5 **The equipment:** Keeping it clean is the most important part. "Whether it's a $50 machine or a $5,000 machine, simply wiping down the parts with a dry paper towel once a week will keep oily buildup from forming," says Riddle.

**Grind beans fresh before each use.

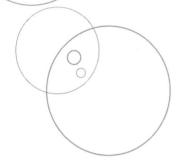

The Ultimate Tea Primer

Everything you need to know about one of the world's healthiest beverages

For most Americans, tea is tea. Forget black teas, white teas, greens, and reds; tea is that finely ground gunpowder that comes in bags from Lipton, or that oversweetened sludge sloshed into plastic bottles and sold in between the Coke and the Mountain Dew. In places like Japan, the UK, and large swaths of Southeast Asia, tea leaves are as diverse and nuanced as wine grapes. Not only does the flavor profile change dramatically between one tea varietal and the next, but so does the caffeine content, the nutritional benefits, and the brewing process.

Regardless of our level of tea sophistication, it's clear we could all benefit from drinking more. Tea has been shown to help ward off everything from heart disease and cancer to bulging waistlines and wrinkles. We've picked the best leaves from around the world and, with the help of a few experts, given you the intel you need to maximize the benefit and the bliss you extract from a simple cup of tea.

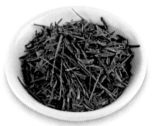

Green Tea

Origins: China, Japan, Southeast Asia

Popular versions: Jasmine Green (a blend of green tea infused with the scent of jasmine flowers), Pin Head Gunpowder, Sencha, Chinese tea, Japanese tea, Dragonwell

Health benefits: Green

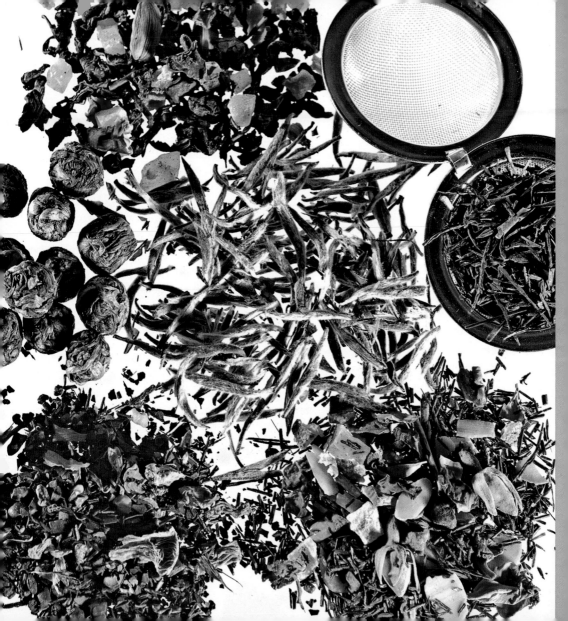

tea has been shown to reduce hypertension, according to a study in the *Archives of Internal Medicine*. People who consumed 120 milliliters of tea every day for at least a year had a 46 percent lower risk of developing hypertension than those who consumed less. Green tea may also help you build a strong skeleton, say scientists in China. They exposed bone cells to tea catechins, which stimulated bone growth and helped slow its breakdown. One of the catechins boosted growth by 79 percent.

Caffeine content: 15–20 milligrams per cup

Brewing tips: For all teas, use one heaping dessert spoonful for every 12 ounces of hot water. Steep green tea leaves in water that's between 165° and 185°F for up to 2½ minutes. "Boiling water scorches tea, which gives it a tart, tannic taste," says Linda Smith, owner and master tea blender at Divinitea.com. "And green tea is an especially sensitive tea leaf." Smith recommends that you bring your pot to a boil, and then remove it from the stove and let it sit for 30 seconds. Steep the leaves for 2 to 2½ minutes. And don't forget to remove the leaves: "The difference between a really good cup and not is to remember to take the tea leaves out—if you leave them in too long, the cup becomes too strong."

Amplify the antioxidants: Add lemon juice to green tea for a huge health boost. When you sip tea, a significant percentage of the polyphenol antioxidants break down before they reach your bloodstream. But researchers at Purdue University discovered that adding lemon juice to the equation helped preserve five times more polyphenols. Squeeze a wedge of lemon into your next cup of hot tea, or try Honest Lemon Black Tea.

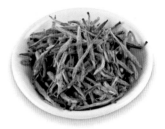

White Tea

Origins: China

Popular versions: Silver Needle, White Peony, Long Life Eyebrow

Health benefit: American researchers found that white tea extract was more effective than green tea extract at fighting bacterial viruses. Additionally, according to a Case Western Reserve University study, an extract of white tea leaves may help fight wrinkles and keep your skin looking young. "Chemicals in the tea appear to protect your skin from sun-induced stress, which can cause the cells to break down and age prematurely," says Elma Baron, MD, the study author. To put white tea to use, try rubbing on a lotion containing white tea extract before you apply your sunblock. Origins A Perfect World White Tea Skin Guardian makes an excellent choice for protection (origins.com, $35).

Caffeine content:
45–60 milligrams per cup

Brewing tips: Steep white tea leaves at 185°F for 3 to 5 minutes. "Americans are used to bigger flavors, but white tea is typically a very delicate taste," Smith says. "If you only leave the leaves in for 2 minutes, you might feel like you're drinking flavored water."

Protect the pearlies:
A study from Temple University found that tea may be the best beverage for your teeth, besides water. Researchers found that teeth immersed in orange juice and soda showed up to five times as much enamel erosion as ones doused in green and black teas. Not only do the drinks contain acids that dissolve enamel, but they also contain sugar.

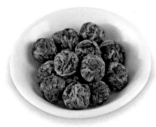

Black Tea

Origins: India, Sri Lanka, Argentina, China

Popular versions:
English Breakfast, Irish Breakfast, Assam, Ceylon, Darjeeling. Earl Grey is a scented black tea made from China black, Ceylon, or India tea, and scented bergamot oil. Chai is also a black tea blend, made from black tea and a variety of spices.

Health benefit: Italian researchers found that drinking 1 cup of black tea per day improves your cardiovascular function—and the more cups you drink, the more you benefit.

A study published in the *Proceedings of the National Academy of Sciences* revealed that drinking 20 ounces of black tea daily causes the body to secrete five times more interferon, a key element of your body's infection-protection arsenal.

Caffeine content:
40–120 milligrams per cup

Brewing tips: Smith recommends that you steep the tea for 3 to 5 minutes in water heated to 185°F, but she is careful to point out that different cultures approach black tea brewing differently. "Every British person I know insists that black tea must be made with boiling water.

"A compromise, then, is to remove the boiling water from the stove for just 10 seconds, rather than 30.

Ditch the dairy:
A study in the *European Heart Journal* found that while black tea can improve blood flow and blood vessel dilation, adding milk to the tea counteracts these effects.

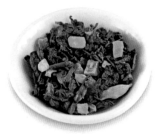

Oolong Tea

Origins: China, Taiwan
Well-known names: Oolong
Health benefit: Japanese scientists found that high levels of antioxidants called polymerized polyphenols, specific to oolong tea, inhibit the body's ability to absorb fat by up to 20 percent. And tea has plenty of other weapons against weight gain. When Taiwanese researchers studied more than 1,100 people over a 10-year period, they determined that those who drank black, green, or oolong tea one or more times a week had nearly 20 percent less body fat than those who drank none. Of course, when the researchers talk about tea, they don't mean the sugary stuff.

Caffeine content: 35–45 milligrams per cup
Brewing tips: Oolong preparation involves a first round of "washing" the tea, which basically means you throw out your first cup. "In China, they wash leaves to wake up the flavor—they believe that the second cup of tea is most flavorful," Smith says. Pour water heated to 185°F over oolong leaves, and let them infuse for 10 seconds. Then remove the leaves, and discard the water. Put the leaves back in, and pour the hot water over top once again. Steep the second cup for 30 seconds to 4 minutes.
Beat back blood pressure: In a 10-year study of more than 1,500 people, scientists at Taiwan's National Cheng Kung University found that drinking at least 4 ounces of oolong tea daily can cut the risk of high blood pressure by 46 percent, and downing more than 20 ounces can slash the risk by a whopping 65 percent.

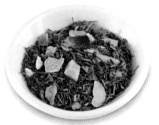

Red Tea

Origins: South Africa
Popular versions: Rooibos, bush tea
Health benefit: Rooibos is loaded with disease-fighting antioxidants and has been shown to boost the immune system. In fact, a recent Japanese study on mice suggests that rooibos tea may help prevent both allergies and cancer.
Caffeine content: 0 milligrams (rooibos is naturally caffeine free)
Brewing tips: Rooibos is a small, needle-like leaf, best used with a fine filter basket or paper filter for those who want a clear cup, Smith says. "A clear cup without any particles leaching through is the preference

of tea drinkers." Just as with all the other varietals, use water heated to 185°F. But only use 1 level teaspoon for every 12 ounces of water and be careful how long you steep, since the flavor can be strong to some. Try out different lengths of time, and decide what flavor suits you best.

Skip the sugar: Rooibos is naturally sweet, so you won't need to add sugar. It's also not technically a tea—it's an herbal infusion.

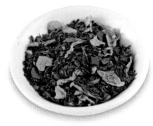

Mate

Origins: South America
Popular versions:
Yerba mate
Caffeine content: Mate contains a caffeine-like sub-stance called mateine. "It's supposed to have a similar effect to caffeine, but without the addiction or jitters," Smith says.

Health benefit: Like green tea on steroids, with up to 90 percent more powerful cancer-fighting antioxidants, a cache of B vitamins, and plenty of chromium, which helps stabilize blood-sugar levels. Plus, its effect on metabolism is so valued that many diet pills list mate as an ingredient.

Brewing tips: Use a tea sack filled with 1 heaping teaspoon of mate for every 12 ounces of water you use. Steep for 1 to 4 minutes.

Drink like a gaucho: In Argentina, yerba mate is consumed out of a hollow gourd filled three-quarters full with the plant, and then covered with water.

Note: For tea's full flavor and nutritional benefits, skip the prebagged stuff and buy loose leaf teas. Pick up all of the varieties in this section from divinitea.com.

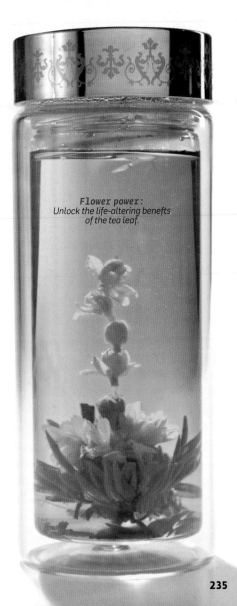

Flower power:
Unlock the life-altering benefts of the tea leaf.

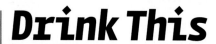

CARIBOU COFFEE

B
Drink Report Card

D+
Food Report Card

• Caribou would be flirting with an A if not for a small cabal of severely over-sugared concoctions holding them back. Between the Coolers and the "wild" menu, there are far too many methods for revving your blood sugar into fat-factory overdrive. The upside is the cappuccinos are as light as they come, and the Northern Lite selections give you plenty of choices to indulge without wrecking your diet.

16

Saturated fat, in grams, in the average medium drink on the Wild menu. That's 80 percent of your day's allowance!

Drink This

Northern Lite Raspberry Latte

(medium, 16.8 fl oz)

130 calories
1 g fat
(0 g saturated)
18 g sugars

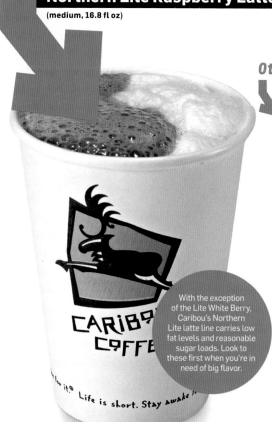

With the exception of the Lite White Berry, Caribou's Northern Lite latte line carries low fat levels and reasonable sugar loads. Look to these first when you're in need of big flavor.

Other Picks

Cappuccino with 2% Milk
(large, 11.9 fl oz)
90 calories
4 g fat
(2.5 g saturated)
9 g sugars

Northern Lite Caramel Cooler
(medium, 20.7 fl oz)
110 calories
2 g fat
(2 g saturated)
14 g sugars

Blended Chai Tea Latte
(small, 16.2 fl oz)
180 calories
3.5 g fat
(2 g saturated)
28 g sugars

520 calories
32 g fat
(19 g saturated)
56 g sugars

Not That!

Lite White Berry Latte

without whip (medium, 12.9 fl oz)

WEAPON OF MASS DESTRUCTION
Large Breve with Whipped Cream
(21.6 fl oz)

710 calories
65 g fat (40 g saturated)
2 g sugars

To order a breve is crazy enough, but to order a large breve is asking for serious trouble. It's a mystery how this drink ever became a café standby. Basically a breve is a latte, but instead of milk, it contains half and half. Now you know the secret to packing 2 days of saturated fat into 1 cup.

Other Passes

Coffee Cooler
(medium, 21.2 fl oz)
320 calories
6 g fat
(6 g saturated)
55 g sugars

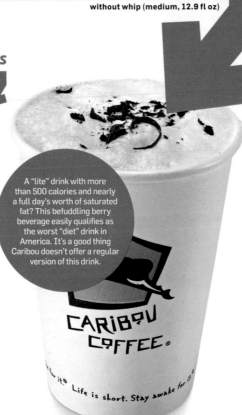

A "lite" drink with more than 500 calories and nearly a full day's worth of saturated fat? This befuddling berry beverage easily qualifies as the worst "diet" drink in America. It's a good thing Caribou doesn't offer a regular version of this drink.

Cookies and Cream Snowdrift
(medium, 23.7 fl oz)
660 calories
23 g fat
(12 g saturated)
89 g sugars

HIDDEN DANGER

Bakery Items at Caribou

From 420-calorie monster cookies to 500-calorie apple fritters, Caribou's food options are exactly the type of sugar-driven carbo catastrophes you should always avoid. The lone star is a simple cup of oatmeal. Everything else, including the reduced-fat items, are trouble.

Passion Fruit Green Tea Smoothie
(small, 17.1 fl oz)
230 calories
0 g fat
52 g sugars

CARIBOU COFFEE®

Life is short. Stay awake for it.®

DUNKIN' DONUTS

A–
Drink
Report
Card

B–
Food
Report
Card

● Despite the long list of indulgent selections, Dunkin' Donuts earns top marks for offering sweet drinks in small, 10-ounce cups and for brewing flavored hot coffees that go way beyond French vanilla. Options such as blueberry, coconut, and toasted almond help you get your flavor fill without pumping your blood full of sugar. Add to that DD's new push toward healthier food options, and you might be able to wrangle yourself a pretty decent meal. Skip the Coolattas and the lattes, steer clear of the bagels and the muffins, and go light on the doughnuts. Follow those rules and you'll have Dunkin' dialed in.

Drink This
Tropicana Orange Coolatta
(small, 16 fl oz)

220 calories
0 g fat
50 g sugars

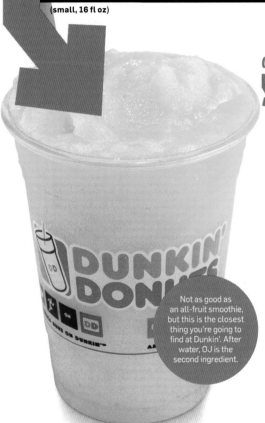

Not as good as an all-fruit smoothie, but this is the closest thing you're going to find at Dunkin'. After water, OJ is the second ingredient.

Other Picks

Raspberry Coffee
(small, 10 fl oz)
15 calories
0 g fat
0 g sugars

Vanilla Latte Lite
(medium, 16 fl oz)
130 calories
0 g fat
15 g sugars

Bavarian Kreme Donut
250 calories
12 g fat
(5 g saturated)
9 g sugars

430 calories
6 g fat
(3.5 g saturated)
86 g sugars

Not That!

Vanilla Bean Coolatta

(small, 16 fl oz)

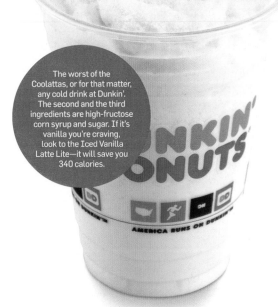

Other Passes

Mocha Raspberry Latte
(small, 10 fl oz)
230 calories
6 g fat
(4 g saturated)
32 g sugars

Vanilla Chai
(14 fl oz)
330 calories
9 g fat
(8 g saturated)
46 g sugars

White Hot Chocolate
(medium, 14 fl oz)
340 calories
13 g fat
(11 g saturated)
45 g sugars

The worst of the Coolattas, or for that matter, any cold drink at Dunkin'. The second and the third ingredients are high-fructose corn syrup and sugar. If it's vanilla you're craving, look to the Iced Vanilla Latte Lite—it will save you 340 calories.

SUGAR SPIKE

Large White Hot Chocolate
(20 fl oz)

The Impact:
63 GRAMS!

When you sweeten your own drinks at home, how many times do you dip the teaspoon into the sugar jar? Two or three? Imagine shoveling in 15 teaspoons, because that's what's happened with this drink. Oh, and it also has 75% of your day's saturated fat.

For 800 calories, you can have

ALL THIS

A Ham, Egg White, and Cheese on Wheat English Muffin; a Glazed Donut; and a Small Vanilla Light Latte

OR

THAT

A Large Coffee Coolatta with Cream

Drink This

Cappuccino

(small, 10 fl oz)

80 calories
4 g fat
(2.5 g saturated)
7 g sugars

HIDDEN DANGER

Honey Bran Raisin Muffin

The bran muffin has long been a symbol of our nutritional miseducation. Its calories come primarily from fat and sugar, making it one of the most overrated foods on the planet. Grab a breakfast sandwich instead.

500 calories
14 g fat
(1.5 g saturated)
48 g sugars

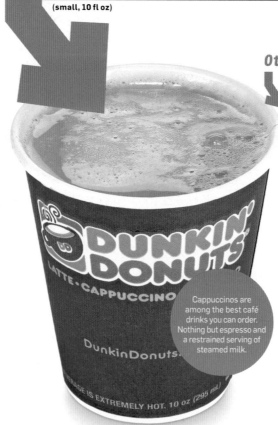

Cappuccinos are among the best café drinks you can order. Nothing but espresso and a restrained serving of steamed milk.

Other Picks

Hazelnut Coffee with Skim Milk and Splenda
(large, 20 fl oz)
45 calories
0 g fat
3 g sugars

Peach Flavored Sweetened Iced Tea
(medium, 16 fl oz)
90 calories
0 g fat
19 g sugars

Bacon, Egg & Cheese Wake-Up Wrap
200 calories
12 g fat
(4.5 g saturated)
620 g sugars

230 calories
11 g fat
(9 g saturated)
24 g sugars

Not That!
Dunkaccino
(small, 10 fl oz)

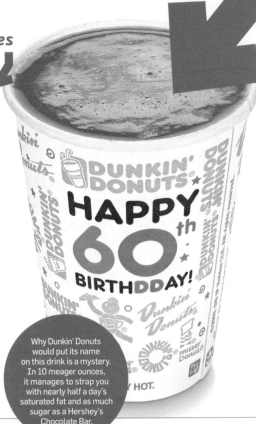

Egg & Cheese on English Muffin
320 calories
13 g fat (5 g saturated)
840 mg sodium

Over the past couple years, DD has made a huge push toward healthier options, and the breakfast sandwiches reflect that effort. In fact, you're guaranteed to keep your sandwich under 400 calories as long as you stick to two rules: Order it on an English muffin and avoid the sausage.

Other Passes

Coffee with Cream and Sugar
(small, 10 fl oz)
120 calories
6 g fat
(4 g saturated)
17 g sugars

Sweet Tea
(medium, 16 fl oz)
120 calories
0 g fat
28 g sugars

Wheat Bagel
(with Reduced Fat Cream Cheese)
450 calories
12 g fat
(5.5 g saturated)
900 g sugars

GUILTY PLEASURE

Mocha Coffee
(medium, 14 fl oz)
170 calories
0 g fat
34 g sugars

Mochas are usually the worst item on a coffee bar menu, but this take on chocolate-spiked caffeine skips the excessive tide of dairy that normally pushes the calorie counts well above the 300 mark. Instead, you get regular joe with a decadent swirl of chocolate and a mild surge of sugar.

Why Dunkin' Donuts would put its name on this drink is a mystery. In 10 meager ounces, it manages to strap you with nearly half a day's saturated fat and as much sugar as a Hershey's Chocolate Bar.

241

STARBUCKS

B-	B
Drink Report Card	Food Report Card

• The best part about Starbucks is the amount of control you have over your order. Switching to fat-free milk and sugar-free syrup can cut massive calories from any drink, but if you fail to specify, you might wind up with more calories than you bargained for. This is especially true if you order one of the nefarious Frappuccinos or flavored espresso drinks. Take the reins and create your own low-calorie tailor-made drink, then throw in one of Starbucks' always-improving food options (some oatmeal, say, or a breakfast wrap) and you're off to a good start to your day.

Drink This

Banana Chocolate Vivanno with Espresso Shot

(grande, 16 fl oz)

270 calories
4.5 g fat
(2 g saturated)
30 g sugars

The Vivannos trump any other frozen drinks on Starbucks' menu. Each one is sweetened with one full banana and fortified with protein and fiber. That makes it a legitimate snack, not just a high-energy treat. And with an espresso shot, you get your breakfast and your morning buzz in a single vessel.

VIVANNO
nourishing blends

Other Picks

Tazo Passion Shaken Iced Green Tea Lemonade
(grande, 16 fl oz)
130 calories
0 g fat
33 g sugars

Nonfat Caramel Macchiato
(tall, 12 fl oz)
140 calories
1 g fat
(0.5 g saturated)
23 g sugars

Caffè Misto
brewed coffee and steamed milk
(venti, 20 fl oz)
130 calories
5 g fat
(3.5 g saturated)
12 g sugars

460 calories
19 g fat
(12 g saturated,
0.5 g trans)
55 g sugars

Not That!

Java Chip Frappuccino Blended Coffee

(grande, 16 fl oz)

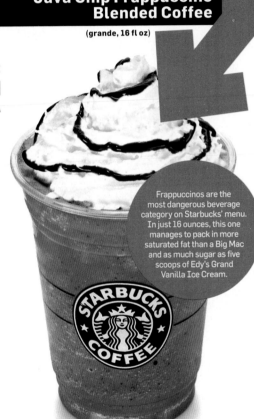

Other Passes

Lemonade Blended Frappuccino

(grande, 16 fl oz)
250 calories
0 g fat
60 g sugars

Nonfat Cinnamon Dolce Latte

(tall, 12 fl oz)
160 calories
0 g fat
30 g sugars

Venti Caffè Latte

(venti, 20 fl oz)
240 calories
9 g fat
(6 g saturated)
22 g sugars

Frappuccinos are the most dangerous beverage category on Starbucks' menu. In just 16 ounces, this one manages to pack in more saturated fat than a Big Mac and as much sugar as five scoops of Edy's Grand Vanilla Ice Cream.

PERFECT PARTNER

Huevos Rancheros Wrap

330 calories
15 g fat (5 g saturated)
610 mg sodium

Want to start your day on nutritionally solid terms? This mock-burrito is guaranteed to fill you up without weighing you down. The secret is in the pairing of eggs with beans, which together provide 16 grams of protein and 8 grams of fiber. Add to that the anti-oxidant jab of roasted peppers and tomatoes and you've got a superlative start to your day.

For 650 calories, you can have

ALL THIS

A Protein Plate, a Vanilla Mini Sparkle Donut, and a Grande Nonfat Tazo Green Tea Latte

OR

THAT

A Venti Green Tea Frappuccino Blended Crème

CALORIE-CUTTING LINGO

HOLD THE WHIP: Cuts the cream and saves you anywhere from 50 to 110 calories

NONFAT: Uses skim milk instead of whole or 2%

SUGAR-FREE SYRUP: Use instead of regular syrup and save up to 150 calories a drink

SKINNY: Tells the barista that you want your drink made with sugar-free syrup and fat-free milk

SIZE MATTERS!

PEPPERMINT WHITE CHOCOLATE MOCHA

VENTI

660 calories

PEPPERMINT WHITE CHOCOLATE MOCHA

tall

496 calories

Total Savings: 164 CALORIES!

Drink This

Venti Caramel Cappuccino

(venti, 20 fl oz)

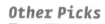

180 calories
4 g fat
(2.5 g saturated)
18 g sugars

If you can put it into words, the Starbucks' staff will be happy to create it. So rather than let an overworked staffer compromise your drink with mindless pumping, just tell them you want a venti 1-pump caramel cappuccino.

Careful, the beverage you're about to enjoy is extremely hot.

Other Picks

Skinny Hazelnut Latte
(grande, 16 fl oz)
110 calories
0g fat
17 g sugars

Iced Skim Vanilla Latte
(grande, 16 fl oz)
200 calories
0 g fat
35 g sugars

Caffé Americano
(venti, 20 fl oz)
25 calories
0 g fat
0 g sugars

320 calories
8 g fat
(5 g saturated)
43 g sugars

Not That!
Venti Caramel Latte
(venti, 20 fl oz)

3.7

The number of miles you'd have to paddle a canoe to burn off the 580 calories in one venti Strawberries and Crème Frappuccino

Other Passes

Hazelnut Signature Hot Chocolate
no whipped cream (grande, 16 fl oz)
480 calories
19 g fat
(11 g saturated)
60 g sugars

Iced White Chocolate Mocha
with 2% milk, no whipped cream (grande, 16 fl oz)
340 calories
9 g fat
(6 g saturated)
52 g sugars

Skim Doubleshot
(venti, 24 fl oz)
150 calories
0 g fat
29 g sugars

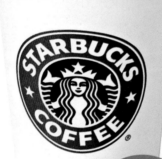

Caramel, vanilla, hazelnut. When it comes to syrup, it's all essentially the same thing: liquid sugar. So expect a similar calorie load no matter which flavors your latte.

Careful, the beverage about to enjoy is extr...

GUILTY PLEASURE

Grande Tazo Vanilla Rooibos Tea Latte
(16 fl oz)
200 calories
5 g fat
(3 g saturated)
31 g sugars

Rooibos is the caffeine-free and antioxidant-rich herb that has been gaining popularity as an alternative to espresso in traditional café drinks. And thanks to its deep, resonant flavor, it makes a pretty good substitution. Give it a shot next time you want something sweet that won't leave you with a case of the Starbucks jitters.

TIM HORTON'S

● Canada's favorite coffee and doughnut dealer is on the march in the US, and that's not such a bad thing for health-conscious caffeine heads. Beyond the respectable line of soups and sandwiches (we can do without the bagels and Timbits) Horton's serves up a solid mix of tea, coffee, and juice. While some espresso drinks are heavy on the sugar, no drink tops the 400-calorie mark.

BEVERAGE MYTH

Iced tea is always a safe play.

Refreshing, teeming with antioxidants, and virtually calorie-free, tea is one of the world's best beverages. The stuff you make at home, anyway. Sweetened restaurant tea has more in common with soda. Tim's 16-ounce Pomegranate Peach White Iced Tea, for instance, is laced with 146 calories from pure sugar—that's as much as a can of Pepsi!

Drink This

Café Mocha
(small, 10 fl oz)

160 calories
7 g fat
(6 g saturated)
21 g sugars

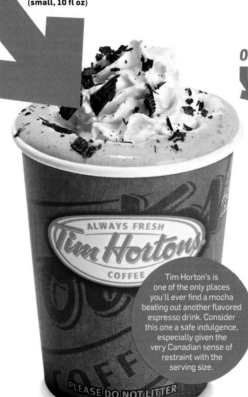

Tim Horton's is one of the only places you'll ever find a mocha beating out another flavored espresso drink. Consider this one a safe indulgence, especially given the very Canadian sense of restraint with the serving size.

Other Picks

Iced Cappuccino with Chocolate Milk
(small, 12 fl oz)
200 calories
1 g fat
(0 g saturated)
44 g sugars

Chocolate Dip Doughnut
210 calories
8 g fat
(3.5 g saturated)
9 g sugars

Tea with Milk and Sugar
(medium, 16 oz)
75 calories
1 g fat
(0.5 g saturated)
14 g sugars

250 calories
8 g fat
(7 g saturated)
31 g sugars

Not That!

French Vanilla Cappuccino

(small, 10 fl oz)

Other Passes

Iced Chocolate Mint Cappuccino Supreme

with cream
(small, 12 fl oz)
390 calories
20 g fat
(13 g saturated)
49 g sugars

Hot Chocolate

(small, 10 oz)
240 calories
6 g fat
(5 g saturated)
38 g sugars

Hot Smoothie

(small, 10 oz)
260 calories
10 g fat
(9 g saturated)
28 g sugars

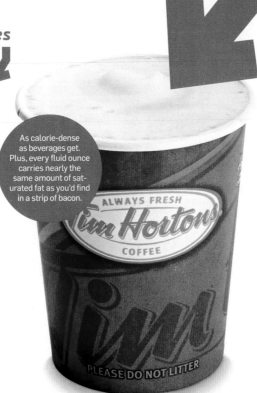

As calorie-dense as beverages get. Plus, every fluid ounce carries nearly the same amount of saturated fat as you'd find in a strip of bacon.

ALWAYS FRESH
Tim Hortons
COFFEE

PLEASE DO NOT LITTER

SUGAR SP★KE

Large Mint Chocolate Chip Cappuccino Supreme

The Impact:
87 G SUGARS!

Imagine dropping 35 Andes Crème de Menthe mints into a warm saucepan, pouring the liquefied chocolate into a cup, and then chugging it. A little sweet? Well that's how much sugar you'll suck down when you order this 20-ounce monstrosity.

PERFECT PARTNER

Chicken Salad Sandwich

380 calories
9 g fat (1 g saturated)
890 mg sodium

Generally "chicken salad" is a euphemism for "chicken-flavored mayonnaise." Tim's version is built with big chunks of white-meat chicken and a light mayo binding for 21 grams of hunger-fighting protein.

247

COFFEE DRINKS
Drink This

No canned coffee will ever beat out a cup of plain joe. In fact, most are littered with more sugar than coffee. Your goal: Get your fix for around 100 calories.

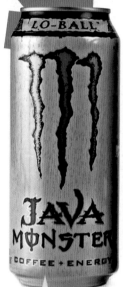

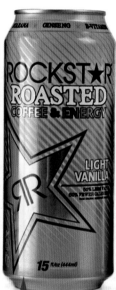

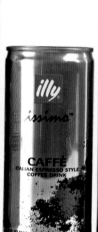

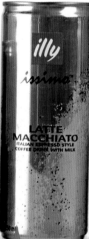

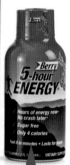

Java Monster Lo-Ball Coffee + Energy
(15 fl oz can)

100 calories
3 g fat
(2 g saturated)
8 g sugars

Delivers the caffeine of a coffee drink with the vitamin load of an energy drink.

Rockstar Roasted Coffee + Energy Light Vanilla
(15 fl oz can)

100 calories
3 g fat
(2 g saturated)
14 g sugars

Contains about two coffee cups' worth of caffeine and a huge dose of B vitamins.

Illy Issimo Caffè
(6.8 fl oz can)

50 calories
0 g fat
(11 g saturated)
11 g sugars

This is by far the best of Illy's canned coffee concoctions. It's light on the calories and heavy on the caffeine.

Illy Issimo Latte Macchiato
(8.45 fl oz can)

110 calories
3 g fat
(0 g saturated)
17 g sugars

Not the best of the Illy line, but even the worst Illy product is better than most other coffee drinks.

5 Hour Energy Berry
(2 fl oz bottle)

4 calories
0 g fat
0 g sugars

This little bottle has as much caffeine as a cup of coffee and a payload of B vitamins that far outperforms the bigger vessels.

Not That!

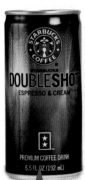

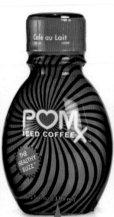

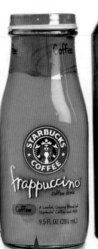

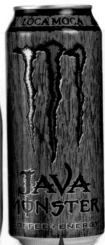

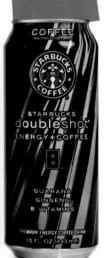

Starbucks Double Shot Espresso and Cream
(6.5 fl oz can)

140 calories
6 g fat
(3.5 g saturated)
17 g sugars

An espresso with cream at a coffee shop will run you about 40 calories.

Pom Café Au Lait Iced Coffee
(10.5 fl oz bottle)

170 calories
3 g fat
(2 g saturated)
20 g sugars

Pom makes great 100% juice products, but their coffee drinks could use a lighter hand with the added sugar.

Starbucks Coffee Frappuccino
(9.5 fl oz bottle)

200 calories
3 g fat
(2 g saturated)
32 g sugars

We'd love to recommend a Starbucks product, but the coffee tycoon has a heavy hand with the sugar.

Java Monster Coffee + Energy Loca Moca
(15 fl oz can)

200 calories
3 g fat
(1 g saturated)
32 g sugars

A morning pickup with more than 10% of your day's calories? Forget it.

Starbucks Coffee Doubleshot Energy + Coffee
(15 fl oz can)

210 calories
2.5 g fat
(1.5 g saturated)
26 g sugars

Starbucks needs to tweak its formula.

Drink This

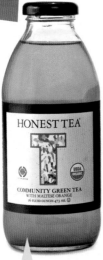

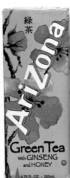

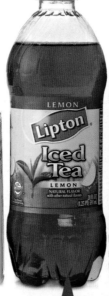

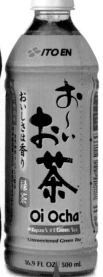

Honest Tea Community Green Tea
(16 fl oz bottle)

34 calories
0 g fat
10 g sugars

High in antioxidants and low in sugar, Honest Tea is one of the most reliable brands in any cooler.

Arizona Green Tea with Ginseng and Honey
(6.75 fl oz box)

45 calories
0 g fat
12 g sugars

One of the few Arizona drinks worth purchasing. Throw this in your work bag for a little antioxidant boost and a light caffeine kick at lunch.

Lipton Lemon Iced Tea
(8 fl oz)

60 calories
0 g fat
16 g sugars

Consider 16 grams your cutoff for sweetened tea. Any more than that and you're facing a nasty blood sugar surge. Buy this in the smallest serving size you can find.

Ito En Oi Ocha Unsweetened Green Tea
(16.9 fl oz)

0 calories
0 g fat
0 g sugars

Researchers believe green tea plays a prominent role in the long lifespans of the Japanese. Ito En is the most popular tea in Japan.

Not That!

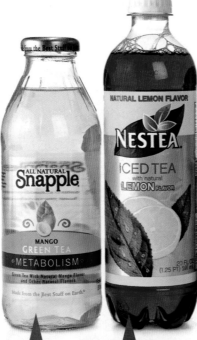

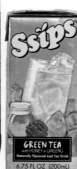

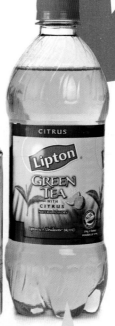

Snapple Mango Green Tea Metabolism
(17.5 fl oz)

140 calories
0 g fat
33 g sugars

Catechins found in green tea can boost metabolism, but whatever metabolic boost you find in this bottle is more than offset by the sugar rush.

Nestea Lemon Iced Tea
(8 fl oz)

80 calories
0 g fat
22 g sugars

Ten calories in each fluid ounce? That's a recipe for weight gain.

Ssips Green Tea with Honey & Ginseng
(6.75 fl oz box)

60 calories
0 g fat
14 g sugars

The honey in the name is just a diversionary tactic. A good part of the sweetness here comes from high-fructose corn syrup. Either way, skip it.

Lipton Green Tea with Citrus
(20 fl oz bottle)

200 calories
0 g fat
53 g sugars

Green tea doesn't actually show up until six ingredients into the list. The first two are water and high-fructose corn syrup.

Drink This

Infusing teas with other liquids (and lots of sugar) has become big business. It can also be a big bust if you don't choose wisely.

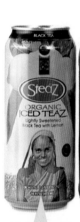

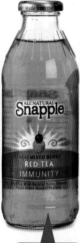

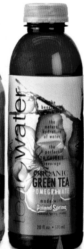

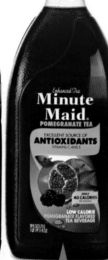

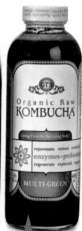

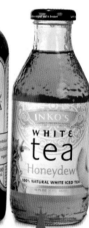

Steaz Organic Iced Teaz Lightly Sweetened with Lemon
(16 fl oz can)

80 calories
0 g fat
20 g sugars

The best tea-lemonade hybrid we've found.

Snapple Red Tea Acai Mixed Berry
(17.5 fl oz bottle)

90 calories
0 g fat
20 g sugars

Red tea is caffeine-free, full of anti-oxidants, and naturally sweeter than other teas.

Arizona Organic Green Tea Pomegranate
(20 fl oz bottle)

50 calories
0 g fat
12.5 g sugars

Arizona's teas are far better than the other beverages put out by the company.

Minute Maid Pomegranate Tea
(8 fl oz)

40 calories
0 g fat
9 g sugars

This is iced tea infused with a 10% blend of apple, pomegranate, and blackberry juices.

GT's Organic Raw Multi-Green Kombucha
(16 fl oz bottle)

70 calories
0 g fat
4 g sugars

Kombucha is Chinese fermented tea, and it's loaded with gut-friendly bacteria.

Inko's White Tea Honeydew
(16 fl oz bottle)

56 calories
0 g fat
14 g sugars

Inko makes a variety of first-rate teas. Like Honest Tea, theirs are naturally flavored and low in sugar.

Not That!

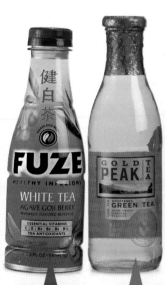

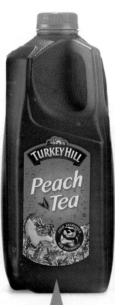

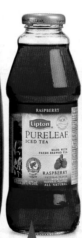

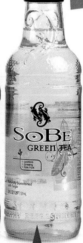

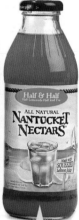

Fuze White Tea Agave Gogi Berry
(18.5 fl oz bottle)

150 calories
0 g fat
37 g sugars

Fuze makes some pretty decent beverages, but this just isn't one of them.

Gold Peak Tea Green Tea
(16.9 fl oz bottle)

170 calories
0 g fat
42 g sugars

Gold Peak would have a decent bottle of tea if it would only cut the sugar by half.

Turkey Hill Peach Tea
(8 fl oz)

100 calories
0 g fat
22 g sugars

This jug contains more sugar than an entire package of Chewy Chips Ahoy cookies.

Lipton PureLeaf Iced Tea Raspberry
(16 fl oz bottle)

150 calories
0 g fat
39 g sugars

If you're going to drink PureLeaf, you should stick to the diet line.

SoBe Green Tea
(20 fl oz bottle)

240 calories
0 g fat
61 g sugars

This bottle has more sugar than six Reese's Peanut Butter Cups. Par for the course for SoBe.

Nantucket Nectars Half and Half
(17.5 fl oz bottle)

190 calories
0 g fat
46 g sugars

Nantucket makes drinks with little to no real fruit and an abundance of added sugar.

8

Drink This, Not That!

WINE

Legend has it that the Benedictine monk Dom Perignon invented champagne in the late 1600s, and announced his discovery by shouting down the halls of the monastery, "Brothers, come quickly! I am drinking stars!"

CHAPTER 8

That's a great story (especially if you happen to own the trademark to "Dom Perignon"). But whether it's true or not, the old monk was most certainly drinking one of the stars of the beverage world. In fact, with each passing year, more and more research points to the health benefits of an occasional glass of fermented grape juice. The latest arrow in wine's quiver is a compound called resveratrol—a substance believed to work on a cellular level, keeping your entire body young and strong. Another substance in wine, saponin, binds to bad cholesterol and ushers it out of the body. And flavonoids—antioxidants that work the same way that vitamins do—can help protect your body against cancer.

Problem is, buying wine or ordering it in a fancy restaurant can feel like an Olympic event—one in which the French judge is holding a grudge against you. Don't let the wine snobs hold you back from getting the health benefits —and the fine, full-bodied flavor—of a nice glass of wine.

Wining without whining

Tip #1: Ignore the label. Really cool labels are designed by marketing companies to unload bad wine on good people. Playful labels with cute animals, cartoons, or bright colors are generally created to sell wine that can't stand on its own.

Tip #2: Shop at the back of the store. Chances are, the bottles close to the counter or featured in the front of the shop are bottles the owner is trying to unload. Either the wine didn't sell as well as expected, or they're getting past their prime. Either way, these won't be among the best bottles in the store.

Tip #3: Forget about the fish/meat

thing. A lot of people get so freaked out by the idea of picking the "wrong" wine to go with their food that they just fall back on the "red meat, red wine" approach. But wines can be mixed and matched with foods much more freely than the sommelier at Le Côte Bastard might let on. Figure out what kind of wines you like, play around with them, and enjoy.

And relax: Dom Perignon was a monk, after all. Whatever wine you choose, trust us: You have his blessing.

How much wine should I be drinking?

Most of us would opt for an after-work visit to the wine bar over a shot of wheatgrass at the juice bar anyday. Thankfully, research continues to show that wine is good for us. The FDA suggests that adults who drink one or two alcoholic beverages a day have the lowest rates of all-cause mortality, and that those who consume moderate amounts of alcohol have a reduced risk of suffering coronary heart disease.

But the threshold between beneficial boozing and detrimental drinking is one you should always be mindful of: Canadian researchers found that, by acting to dilate blood vessels,

a single drink of red wine or other alcohol allows your heart to work less. However, the second drink was found to increase heart rate and blood flow without additional dilation, causing researchers to warn that repeated high consumption can lead to higher risk of heart attacks. A separate study from the Medical University of South Carolina found that middle-age nondrinkers who started consuming moderate amounts of alcohol (one drink a day for women, two drinks for men) had a 38 percent lower chance of developing cardiovascular disease after 4 years than their nondrinking counterparts. Don't be determined to finish the bottle when a glass will do.

Most Americans select their wine by grape variety, turning to familiar names such as chardonnay and cabernet sauvignon. This makes perfect sense because a grape variety (grapes are "varieties"; the wines named for them are "varietals") has the single biggest impact on a wine's flavor. It's the wine equivalent of choosing chocolate, vanilla, or strawberry. This primer introduces the wine grape varieties that Americans reach for most. It will help you to identify wines that suit your taste, your budget, and your dinner.

Wine Glossary

Simplifying the sometimes stupefying world of wine terminology

AROMA All that glass swirling and sniffing isn't just for show. The flavor of a wine, as with other foods, is the result of your taste and smell combined, making aroma an important part of the experience. Some wine grapes are only lightly aromatic, while a few, like Viognier, can smell like imposter perfume. It's all about preference.

BODY Think of body as weighing the wine on your tongue. Water is light bodied; cream is heavy bodied; the various milk iterations fall somewhere in between. When matching wine to food, choosing a wine with a similar weight, or body, is usually the best place to start.

RESVERATROL Wine contains many compounds that have been shown to have health benefits in moderation, including the ethanol, or alcohol, itself. Resveratrol, found in the skins and seeds of grapes, may help prevent cancer, viral infections, and heart disease. Some varieties have more than others.

TANNIN Tannin is found primarily in red wines because they have prolonged contact with grape skins and seeds where tannins are found naturally. You can sense tannins on your palate as a dry, sometimes gritty, sensation similar to drinking black tea.

DRY Dry simply means a wine is without detectable sweetness. Dry wines have less than 2 grams of sugar/liter in them (referred to as residual sugar) and many dry reds have less than 1 gram. However, a demi-sec champagne may have as much as 50 grams/liter. A wine with a hint of sweetness can be called off-dry.

VINTAGE Simply, the year the grapes were grown for a wine is called its vintage, which is usually expressed by a date on the label. Because grapes are affected by weather, some years are better than others, resulting in good and poor vintages.

FINISH This is what's left after you swallow the wine, including the types of flavors and how long they last in your mouth.

Pinot Grigio

When it comes to Italian cuisine, Americans live by the three p's—pizza, pasta, and pinot grigio, the top-selling imported wine in the United States.

Actually a mutation of the red grape pinot noir, pinot grigio appears in France under the name pinot gris. (Same grape—two very different wines.) The Italian pinot grigio usually denotes a light, crisp white, while pinot gris sticks closer to its red grape roots, rich and fuller-bodied with pear and spice flavors.

Aroma	Low to medium
Body	Light to full
Acidity	Medium to high
Aging Potential	None to short-term (5 years)
Resveratrol	Very low

EVERYDAY EXCELLENCE

Woodbridge Pinot Grigio

2009, California; $7

Wow! Plenty of body, pear and spice, all for the price of an Extra-Value Meal.

WEEKEND WARRIOR

Collavini Pinot Grigio Villa Canlungo Black Label DOC Collio

2008, Italy; $19

Like diving into a swimming pool of pineapple and apple juice, then getting snapped by a wet towel.

BLOWOUT BUY

Domaine Marc Kreydenweiss Moenchberg Pinot Gris Alsace Grand Cru

2007, France; $55

Sweet apricot balanced with crisp acidity and wet stone.

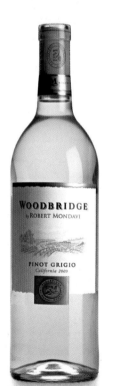

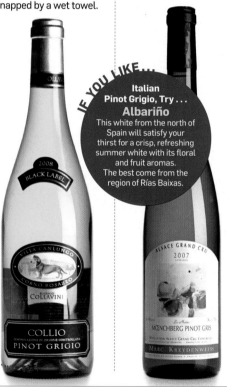

IF YOU LIKE...

Italian Pinot Grigio, Try ...
Albariño
This white from the north of Spain will satisfy your thirst for a crisp, refreshing summer white with its floral and fruit aromas. The best come from the region of Rías Baixas.

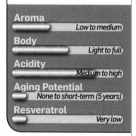

Pinot Grigio: 3 Ways

Italy Most Italian pinot grigios come from the cool northern regions. They're chuggable whites that can be kept in the fridge, ready to pop open on the beach or in place of a beer on a hot summer day.

Drink This! **Bottega Vinaia Pinot Grigio** *2008, Italy; $18*

Alsace If Italian pinot grigio resembles spring water with lemon, the Alsatian stuff slugs down more like a banana milk shake, creamy and rich, with flavors of apple, pear, apricot, and, yes, banana, along with occasional smoke and spice.

Drink This! **Helfrich Pinot Gris** *2007, Alsace, France; $15*

Oregon Until 2007, Oregon made only pinot gris. The state didn't recognize the term pinot grigio for wine labels. Just as well because these wines generally lean toward the richer, fuller French style.

Drink This! **WillaKenzie Estate Pinot Gris, Willamette Valley** *2008, Oregon; $18*

Drink This
Alois Lageder Pinot Grigio Dolomiti
Alto Adige, Italy 2008; $17

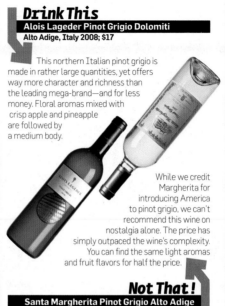

This northern Italian pinot grigio is made in rather large quantities, yet offers way more character and richness than the leading mega-brand—and for less money. Floral aromas mixed with crisp apple and pineapple are followed by a medium body.

While we credit Margherita for introducing America to pinot grigio, we can't recommend this wine on nostalgia alone. The price has simply outpaced the wine's complexity. You can find the same light aromas and fruit flavors for half the price.

Not That!
Santa Margherita Pinot Grigio Alto Adige
2008; $22

Pinot Grigio-Friendly Foods

With a body that ranges from anemic to Ah-nold, pinot grigio (aka gris) can pair with light seafood or wild game depending on its style. In most cases, however, you'll be drinking the lighter, more available grigio.

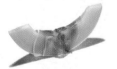

BEST SNACK
Melon with proscuitto

BEST TAKE-OUT
Sushi

BEST DINNER PARTY
Pasta with fruit de mer

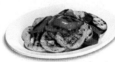

BEST COOKOUT
Grilled summer vegetables

Sauvignon Blanc

● Easily one of the most characterful and explosive of the popular varietal wines, sauvignon blanc has a variety of styles, all of which include intense aromas and acidity that hit your palate like a kiss from a light socket.

The flavors range from tart, minerally, and smoky in its home in France's Loire Valley, to tropical with notes of citrus in California (where it's often called fume blanc), or grassy and herbal in New Zealand, where this single grape makes up 75 percent of all wine exports.

Aroma — High
Body — Light to medium
Acidity — High
Aging Potential — None to short-term (5 years)
Resveratrol — Very low

EVERYDAY EXCELLENCE
Brancott Sauvignon Blanc
2009, New Zealand; $13

Light-bodied, zesty, and electric with big flavor of grapefruit soda.

WEEKEND WARRIOR
Sauvion & Fils Sancerre
2008; $28

Like lightly salted celery, with green berry and herb garden flavors.

BLOWOUT BUY
Robert Mondavi Fumé Blanc Reserve To Kalon
2007, California; $40

An oaked, yet balanced style, with rich flavors of fig, pineapple, and vanilla.

IF YOU LIKE...

Sauvignon Blanc, Try...
Verdejo
This grape, found in the white wines of Spain's Rueda region, makes crisp and aromatic white wines. Their citrus fruit and occasional grassiness draw comparisons to sauvignon blanc.

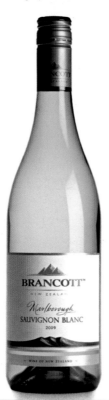

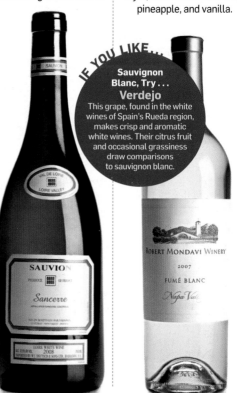

Sauvignon Blanc: 3 Ways

Loire Valley Flavors of gun smoke and gooseberries are considered a good thing in these occasionally outrageous wines. The limestone soils of Sancerre and Poully-Fumé can give the wine whiffs of a chalkboard eraser.
***DRINK THIS!* Remy Pannier Sancerre** *2007; $24*

New Zealand Get your salad fork ready. The sauvignon blanc that put New Zealand on the wine map can be like rummaging through the crisper drawer, with vegetal flavors of green bell pepper, spring peas, asparagus, and chives.
***DRINK THIS!* Nobilo Sauvignon Blanc Marlborough** *2008, New Zealand; $13*

California In warmer climates, like Cali, sauvignon blanc goes into tropical vacation mode, with a whallop of pink grapefruit, guava, and passion fruit.
***DRINK THIS!* Hanna Sauvignon Blanc Russian River Valley** *2008, California; $18*

Drink This
Viña Montes Sauvignon Blanc Leyda Valley
2008, Chile; $16

Leyda Valley is quickly becoming recognized as one of the top spots for sauvignon blanc, capturing everything the grape has to offer, from citrus fruit to minerals and the sweet pea and herb flavors that go missing in warmer climates.

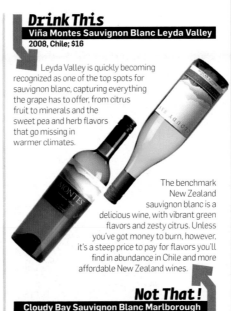

The benchmark New Zealand sauvignon blanc is a delicious wine, with vibrant green flavors and zesty citrus. Unless you've got money to burn, however, it's a steep price to pay for flavors you'll find in abundance in Chile and more affordable New Zealand wines.

Not That!
Cloudy Bay Sauvignon Blanc Marlborough
2008, New Zealand; $27

Sauvignon Blanc-Friendly Foods

If ever there were a wine for vegetarians, it's sauvignon blanc. The crisp, vegetal flavors make this the go-to wine for stump-the-sommelier foods such as asparagus and artichokes.

BEST SNACK
Edamame

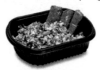

BEST TAKEOUT
Middle Eastern

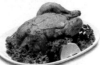

BEST DINNER PARTY
Roast chicken with lemon

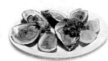

BEST COOKOUT
Raw oysters

WINE INSIDER
Pyra-Maniac

If your sauvignon blanc smells like a celery stick, it's due to pyrazines—a class of potent chemicals that give off green aromas. Methoxypyrazines, found in sauvignon blanc, are the same compounds that lend their distinct flavors to bell peppers, peas, and beets.

DRINK TO YOUR HEALTH
Protect and Serve

Polyphenols reside in grape skins, which are used in making red wine but are removed when making white. However, new research shows that the flesh of grapes, used in white wine, may offer the same cardio protection as the skins. A study published in the *Journal of Agricultural and Food Chemistry* found that giving white wine to rats both protected against heart attack and aided in recovery following an attack.

Chardonnay

Like milk, bread, and eggs, chardonnay is an American grocery staple—outselling all other varietal wines. Fortunately for us, there is plenty to go around because chardonnay is planted practically everywhere that wine grapes grow. For this reason, it can be a difficult wine to pin down. One minute it's all lean, crisp, and acidic, as in chablis, then it's plush, tropical, and buttery when grown in warmer climates and aged in oak. Maybe the versatility is why we love chard so dearly.

Aroma	
	Low to medium
Body	
	Medium to full
Acidity	
	Low to high
Aging Potential	
None to mid-term (5 to 10 years)	
Resveratrol	
	Very low

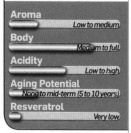

EVERYDAY EXCELLENCE
Veramonte Chardonnay Casablanca Valley Reserva
2008, Chile; $11

Rich and lush for the price, with tropical fruit and spicy oak.

WEEKEND WARRIOR
Chappellet Chardonnay Napa Valley
2008, California; $30

Ripe pear and figgy fruit with aromas of Mom's apple pie on the windowsill.

BLOWOUT BUY
Louis Jadot Puligny-Montrachet
2007; $50

Complex toast and mineral nuances with a long hazelnut finish.

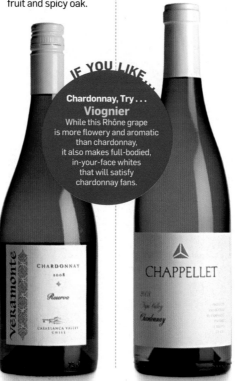

IF YOU LIKE...

Chardonnay, Try . . . Viognier
While this Rhône grape is more flowery and aromatic than chardonnay, it also makes full-bodied, in-your-face whites that will satisfy chardonnay fans.

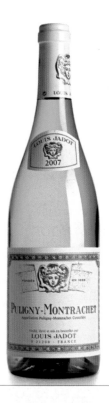

Chardonnay: 3 Ways

Australia South Eastern Australia makes boatloads of chardonnay, most of which sail directly to America. Wines labeled "unoaked" or "naked" indicate crisper wines with no oak aging.
***DRINK THIS!* Yellow Tail Chardonnay, The Reserve** *2007, South Eastern Australia; $11*

Burgundy The classic regions of Chablis, Meursault, Chassagne-Montrachet, and Puligny-Montrachet require both a pronunciation guide and a fat wallet. These are the original chardonnays, complex in flavor and able to age.
***DRINK THIS!* Louis Jadot Meursault** *2006, France; $50*

Napa Valley This is where the over-the-top, butter-bomb style of chardonnay emerged—the California wine equivalent of '80s big hair. While most Cali wines strive for balance these days, they still tend to be heavy on oak and alcohol.
***DRINK THIS!* Acacia Carneros Chardonnay** *California; $22*

Drink This
Hardys Chardonnay South Eastern Australia
2009; $7

The Aussies are unbeatable when it comes to making mass quantities of tasty chardonnay. The spiced apple flavors in this bargain bottle are crisp with just enough sweet oak. Buy the same wine by the 3-liter box and bring your price below 5 bucks a "bottle"!

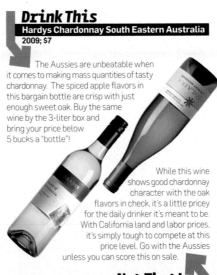

While this wine shows good chardonnay character with the oak flavors in check, it's a little pricey for the daily drinker it's meant to be. With California land and labor prices, it's simply tough to compete at this price level. Go with the Aussies unless you can score this on sale.

Not That!
Robert Mondavi Chardonnay
Santa Lucia Highlands Solaire
2007; $15

Chardonnay-Friendly Foods

As a full-bodied white, chardonnay is a classic pairing for poultry and seafood. With big body, a creamy texture, and good acidity, chardonnay also plays well with butter and cream sauces.

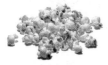
BEST SNACK
Popcorn

BEST TAKEOUT
Fish and chips

BEST DINNER PARTY
Pasta with Alfredo sauce

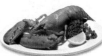
BEST COOKOUT
Steamed lobster

Pinot Noir

● Having trouble finding an affordable pinot noir? Blame Hollywood! According to economists, the 2004 movie *Sideways* completely reversed the wine's falling price, with the most dramatic increase in $20 to $40 wines.

While it has the lightest body and tannins of the classic red grapes, it can possess a haunting variety of flavors: berries, cola, tea, mushroom, even hints of barnyard. As the lead character Miles eloquently observed, there is something magical about pinot noir.

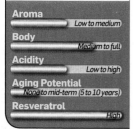

Aroma	Low to medium
Body	Medium to full
Acidity	Low to high
Aging Potential	None to mid-term (5 to 10 years)
Resveratrol	High

EVERYDAY EXCELLENCE
Arrogant Frog Lilly Pad Noir
2008, Vin de Pays d'Oc, France; $10

Earthy and dark, with ripe raspberry and smoked sausage notes.

WEEKEND WARRIOR
Sokol Blosser Pinot Noir Dundee Hills
2007, Oregon; $40

Tastes like cherry cola for adults, with a smooth, supple finish.

BLOWOUT BUY
Chanson Pére & Fils Pernand-Vergelesses Les Vergelesses
2005, Burgundy, France; $62

Sour cherry pie with baking spices, licorice, and fine, silky tannins.

IF YOU LIKE...
Pinot Noir, Try ...
Cru Beaujolais
Beaujolais is made in Burgundy, not from pinot noir but from the gamay grape. The top crus, or regions, including Fleurie and Morgon, make light-bodied reds resembling basic Burgundy for about $20.

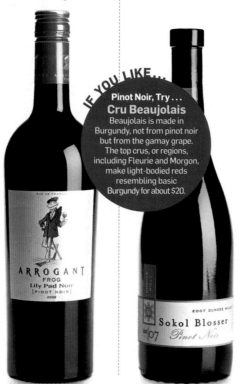

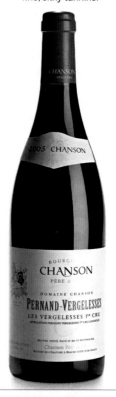

Pinot Noir: 3 Ways

Red Burgundy These wines rarely say pinot noir on the label, preferring to list their fancy French region or vineyard. Generally light-bodied and supple, the best display the complexity and finesse that give pinot its sexy reputation.

DRINK THIS! **Bouchard Père & Fils Bourgogne Rouge Reserve** *2007, Burgundy, France; $24*

Oregon Pinot is Oregon's top grape, but small wineries means it doesn't come cheap. These wines are frequently $40 or more, but at their best can compete with the pricier Burgundies.

DRINK THIS! **Ponzi Tavola Pinot Noir Willamette Valley** *2007, Oregon; $25*

California Ready to jump at any trend, California has cranked up pinot production. The best come from cooler areas like the Russian River Valley and Sonoma Coast.

DRINK THIS! **BearBoat Pinot Noir Russian River Valley** *2007; $20*

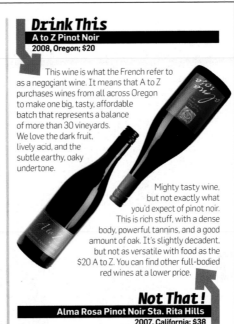

Drink This
A to Z Pinot Noir
2008, Oregon; $20

This wine is what the French refer to as a negociant wine. It means that A to Z purchases wines from all across Oregon to make one big, tasty, affordable batch that represents a balance of more than 30 vineyards. We love the dark fruit, lively acid, and the subtle earthy, oaky undertone.

Mighty tasty wine, but not exactly what you'd expect of pinot noir. This is rich stuff, with a dense body, powerful tannins, and a good amount of oak. It's slightly decadent, but not as versatile with food as the $20 A to Z. You can find other full-bodied red wines at a lower price.

Not That!
Alma Rosa Pinot Noir Sta. Rita Hills
2007, California; $38

Pinot Noir-Friendly Foods

If pinot noir were in grade school, the teacher would give it a gold star for "gets along well with others." This light-bodied red is a peacemaker at any dinner table, able to handle meat, poultry, and flavorful fish with ease.

BEST SNACK
Chips with black bean dip

BEST TAKEOUT
Chinese

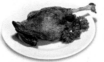

BEST DINNER PARTY
Roast duck

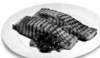

BEST COOKOUT
Grilled salmon steaks

Temp Tenets

Most wines—both red and white—taste their best around 55°F, but you may want to serve crisp whites such as riesling and sauvignon blanc slightly (5°-8°) colder, and full-bodied reds such as merlot and cabernet sauvignon slightly (5°-8°) warmer. Remember the 20-minute rule: White wines should be taken out of the fridge 20 minutes before serving to warm, just as reds should be put in 20 minutes before serving to chill.

DRINK TO YOUR HEALTH

Pinot Power

Multiple studies have demonstrated that pinot noir consistently contain the highest levels of resveratrol among wines. One study found that pinot had more than five times the amount found in California cabernet sauvignon.

Zinfandel

● Zinfandel is as American as Levis and bank bailouts. Like all red wines, it gets its red color from grape juice coming in contact with the skins. In the 1980s, wine-makers left the wine on the skins only briefly to create a sweet, pink wine they dubbed white zinfandel, although it is made from the same red grapes. Now it's white zinfandel, rather than the red stuff, that leads the way in consumption. But whether you like it white and sweet, or red and peppery, zin is worth exploring.

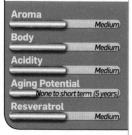

Aroma	
	Medium
Body	
	Medium
Acidity	
	Medium
Aging Potential	
None to short term (5 years)	
Resveratrol	
	Medium

EVERYDAY EXCELLENCE
Rancho Zabaco Dancing Bull Winemaker's Reserve Zinfandel
2007, California; $10

Like a shopping cart collision in the jelly aisle—a berry explosion.

WEEKEND WARRIOR
Artezin Zinfandel, Mendocino County
2007, California; $18

Pretty plum meets baking spices and hints of licorice.

BLOWOUT BUY
Dashe Zinfandel, Dry Creek Valley
2008, California; $24

Like a vanilla sundae drizzled with cherry topping—jammy, gooey fruit goodness.

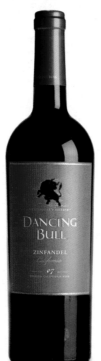

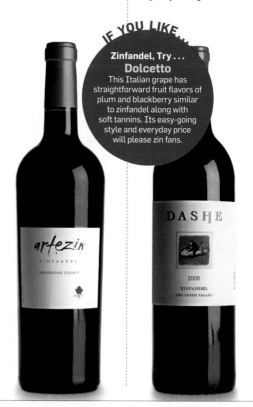

IF YOU LIKE...

Zinfandel, Try ...
Dolcetto
This Italian grape has straightforward fruit flavors of plum and blackberry similar to zinfandel along with soft tannins. Its easy-going style and everyday price will please zin fans.

Zinfandel: 3 Ways

California Zinfandel The majority of America's 50,000 acres of zin are sprawled along the California coast. Zinfandel has the type of raspberry fruit you find in a jar of jam, with licorice and herbs, high alcohol, and low tannins.

DRINK THIS! **Ravenswood Vintners Blend Zinfandel** *2007, California; $10*

Italian Primitivo Most prominent in Puglia (picture the heel of the Italian boot), these wines are called both primitivo and zinfandel. They're generally lighter in body and alcohol than their California cousins and rarely top 20 bucks.

DRINK THIS! **Li Veli "Orion" Primitivo** *2007, Italy; $11*

White Zinfandel A rosé in color but smells and tastes considerably sweeter. While most dry red wines have less than 2 g/liter of sugar, white zinfandels have about twice that amount.

DRINK THIS! **Buehler Vineyards Napa Valley White Zinfandel** *2007, California; $7*

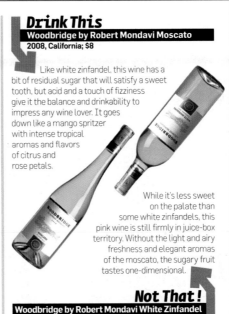

Drink This
Woodbridge by Robert Mondavi Moscato
2008, California; $8

Like white zinfandel, this wine has a bit of residual sugar that will satisfy a sweet tooth, but acid and a touch of fizziness give it the balance and drinkability to impress any wine lover. It goes down like a mango spritzer with intense tropical aromas and flavors of citrus and rose petals.

While it's less sweet on the palate than some white zinfandels, this pink wine is still firmly in juice-box territory. Without the light and airy freshness and elegant aromas of the moscato, the sugary fruit tastes one-dimensional.

Not That!
Woodbridge by Robert Mondavi White Zinfandel
2009, California; $7

Sweet Sipping

All wines contain sugar. A small amount is always left over following fermentation, and some may be added by the winemaker, as it is with champagne. Many wine labels now list the residual sugar, usually indicated in grams/liter.

Most dry wines have between 1 and 2 grams of residual sugar, which doesn't taste sweet at all. Above 2 grams and you may start to sense sweet flavors, making the wine either "off-dry" or "semi-sweet." Wines with more than 45 g/l are considered sweet, and some of the world's best dessert wines, like sauternes, can contain hundreds of grams per liter. While this sounds like little more than a dental nightmare, sugar doesn't exist by itself in a wine. By tempering the sweetness with acidity, the best sweet wines achieve liveliness and balance without seeming cloying.

Zinfandel-Friendly Foods

With its obvious sweetness, white zinfandel goes well with spicy foods, while the red stuff, with its big berry flavors and medium tannins, is great with tomato dishes and comfort foods like Thanksgiving turkey.

BEST SNACK
Barbecue potato chips

BEST TAKEOUT
Mexican

BEST DINNER PARTY
Eggplant parmesan

BEST COOKOUT
Burgers

Syrah

Syrah is a grape with two different identities, the stately syrah of France's Rhône region and the sassy Australian stuff that prefers to go by shiraz. The best of French syrah (often labeled Cote-Rotie, Hermitage, or Côtes du Rhône) can be dark and intense, with mineral, pepper, bacon, leather, and tobacco flavors. In a word: rustic.

The shiraz of Australia and South Africa tend to be ripe and friendly with blueberry and hints of pepper. In the US, syrah does well in California and Washington.

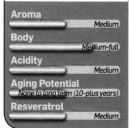

Aroma
Medium

Body
Medium-full

Acidity
Medium

Aging Potential
None to long term (10-plus years)

Resveratrol
Medium

EVERYDAY EXCELLENCE
Jacob's Creek Reserve Shiraz
2006, South Australia; $12

Easy-drinking, smooth, and juicy with mixed berry fruit.

WEEKEND WARRIOR
Vidal-Fleury Crozes Hermitage
2007; $24

Like a black plum with an iron nail sticking out of it, firm with good acidity.

BLOWOUT BUY
Viña Montes Folly Santa Cruz
2006, Chile; $90

Biting into a chocolate filled with Starbucks coffee and blackberry jam. Decadent!

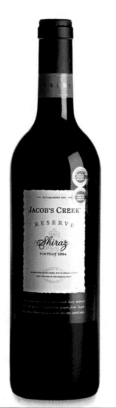

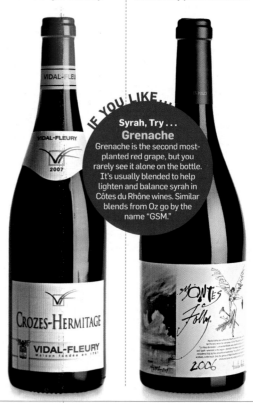

IF YOU LIKE...

Syrah, Try ... Grenache
Grenache is the second most-planted red grape, but you rarely see it alone on the bottle. It's usually blended to help lighten and balance syrah in Côtes du Rhône wines. Similar blends from Oz go by the name "GSM."

Syrah: 3 Ways

Rhône Red In the northern Rhône, syrah stands alone, while in the south it plays backup in blends. Rhône syrahs tend to be dark and intense, with iron and meat flavors, as well as softer violet and berry aromas.

DRINK THIS! **M. Chapoutier Crozes-Hermitage La Petite Ruche** *2007; $25*

Australian Shiraz More bountiful than kangaroos in Oz. The juicy, blueberry-flavored budget wines come from the huge region called South Australia. Barossa Valley and McLaren Vale are prestigious regions with prices to match.

DRINK THIS! **Woop Woop Shiraz** *2008, Australia; $12*

American Syrah It's not cab or merlot, but syrah has serious devotees along California's Central Coast. Washington is a new and promising area for syrah, but most start at $30 or more.

DRINK THIS! **Zaca Mesa Syrah, Santa Ynez Valley** *2005, California; $20*

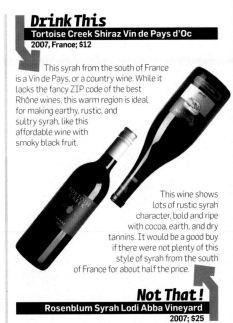

Drink This
Tortoise Creek Shiraz Vin de Pays d'Oc
2007, France; $12

This syrah from the south of France is a Vin de Pays, or a country wine. While it lacks the fancy ZIP code of the best Rhône wines, this warm region is ideal for making earthy, rustic, and sultry syrah, like this affordable wine with smoky black fruit.

This wine shows lots of rustic syrah character, bold and ripe with cocoa, earth, and dry tannins. It would be a good buy if there were not plenty of this style of syrah from the south of France for about half the price.

Not That!
Rosenblum Syrah Lodi Abba Vineyard
2007; $25

Syrah-Friendly Foods

As a serious red wine, syrah likes serious red meat. The smoky and gamey flavors found in French syrah make it a favorite with lamb, grilled meats, and stews.

BEST SNACK
Beef jerky

BEST TAKEOUT
Gyro

BEST DINNER PARTY
Rack of lamb

BEST COOKOUT
Grilled sausages

Is Organic Better?

Clearly, choosing organic wine is a good idea for the planet and local communities, but does it really make a difference in terms of your health? According to a 2006 study appearing in the *Journal of Agricultural and Food Chemistry* that compared organic and nonorganic syrah grapes as they ripened, the level of anthocyanins, which have been shown to fight cancer, were actually higher in the conventionally grown grapes, not the organic. If you are allergic to sulfites, a condition that affects about 1 percent of the population, organic wines can be a good choice because they do not have added sulfites. But in general, while organic producers may try to imply your health is at stake, it has not been proven that organic wines offer health benefits over conventional wines.

271

Merlot

It's tough to love cabernet and not love merlot, too. As brothers from Bordeaux, merlot's softer plum, cherry, and coffee flavors are used to balance the more rigid cabernet in classic Bordeaux blends.

In California, these blends sometimes go by the name meritage. Still not convinced? You've probably enjoyed a cab-merlot blend without even realizing it. Often a little cabernet finds its way into a wine labeled merlot and vice versa, as a way to add balance and complexity.

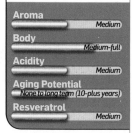

Aroma	
	Medium
Body	
	Medium-full
Acidity	
	Medium
Aging Potential	
None to long term (10-plus years)	
Resveratrol	
	Medium

EVERYDAY EXCELLENCE
Falesco Merlot
2007, Umbria; $12

Soft as a baby's blanket, with rich cherry and sweet vanilla flavors.

WEEKEND WARRIOR
Casa Lapostolle Merlot Cuvée Alexandre Apalta Vineyard Merlot
2007, Chile; $18

No wimpy merlot, this is dark stuff with chocolate, chewy fruit, and fine tannins.

BLOWOUT BUY
Plumpjack Napa Valley Merlot
2007; $50

Ready to take on any cabernet with copious notes of coffee and chocolate-covered cherries.

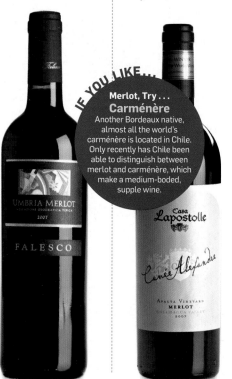

IF YOU LIKE...

Merlot, Try ...
Carménère
Another Bordeaux native, almost all the world's carménère is located in Chile. Only recently has Chile been able to distinguish between merlot and carménère, which make a medium-boded, supple wine.

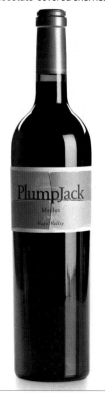

Merlot: 3 Ways

Red Bordeaux While much of the Bordeaux merlot, like Château Pétrús, are rare and expensive, not all Bordeaux has to be pricey. Good vintages like 2005 offer amazing values.

DRINK THIS! **Christian Moueix Encore Merlot** *2005, Bordeaux, France; $15*

American Merlot California deserves the rap for introducing Americans to thin, stalky-tasting, cheap merlot, but there are also great wines made there. In addition, merlot is heavily planted in Washington and New York's Long Island.

DRINK THIS! **Hogue Genesis Merlot** *2006, Columbia Valley; $10*

Southern Hemisphere In South America, merlot is grown in Argentina but performs especially well in Chile. In Australia, merlot is far less popular than shiraz, but the west coast makes excellent merlot and cabernet.

DRINK THIS! **Lapostolle Casa Merlot, Rapel Valley** *2007, Chile; $14*

Drink This
Yellow Tail Merlot South Eastern Australia
2009; $8

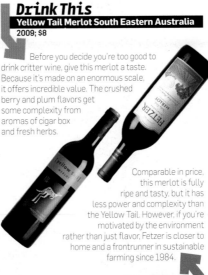

Before you decide you're too good to drink critter wine, give this merlot a taste. Because it's made on an enormous scale, it offers incredible value. The crushed berry and plum flavors get some complexity from aromas of cigar box and fresh herbs.

Comparable in price, this merlot is fully ripe and tasty, but it has less power and complexity than the Yellow Tail. However, if you're motivated by the environment rather than just flavor, Fetzer is closer to home and a frontrunner in sustainable farming since 1984.

Not That!
Fetzer Merlot California Valley Oaks
2007; $9

To Decant or Not to Decant?

It sounds fancy, but decanting is nothing more than carefully pouring a wine from its bottle into a glass container for serving. There are two primary reasons to decant wine, and merlot suits them both.

Decant aged reds: After a decade in the bottle, most powerful red wines may leave some sediment in the bottle. By carefully decanting the wine, you can leave the sludge behind.

Decant young reds: Some powerful red wines can be tight when they are young. It's as if the wine is holding on to its aromas and flavors with a vice grip. Decanting aerates the wine and releases more flavors.

Lastly, decant box wines. There are now good quality, affordable wines available in boxes, but stigmas still get in the way. Pouring it from a nice glass vessel will solve that.

Merlot-Friendly Foods

With its red fruit and black fruit, full-bodied merlot can handle grilled red meat, while lighter versions are a good choice with poultry or even pasta. The mocha and earthy flavors also work well with mushrooms.

BEST SNACK
Dark chocolate

BEST TAKEOUT
Fried chicken

BEST DINNER PARTY
Spaghetti and meatballs

BEST COOKOUT
Grilled portabella caps

Cabernet Sauvignon

● Cabernet is like the high-school quarterback of red grapes: muscular, charismatic, and incredibly popular. Whether bottled alone or in a blend, cabernet brings complexity and power. Its abundance of tannins and generous mouth feel make this a wine that can handle the heartiest foods. And the best cabs are built to last. With inky dark fruit, such as black cherry and cassis, as well as spicy and herbal flavors of mint and eucalyptus, this grape knows how to wow a crowd.

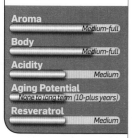

Aroma	Medium-full
Body	Medium-full
Acidity	Medium
Aging Potential	None to long term (10-plus years)
Resveratrol	Medium

EVERYDAY EXCELLENCE
Nieto Senetiner Cabernet Sauvignon Reserva Mendoza
2008, Argentina; $11

Lots of power for the price, a mix of blackberry with vanilla beans and toast.

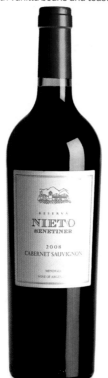

WEEKEND WARRIOR
Louis M. Martini Cabernet Sauvignon Sonoma County
2007; $17

Like opening a dusty cedar chest to find it's filled with plums and chocolate bars. Score!

BLOWOUT BUY
Duckhorn Vineyards Cabernet Sauvignon Napa Valley
2006; $65

Crushed red fruit and super-fine tannins that buff your tongue like fine sandpaper.

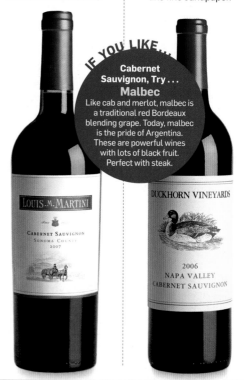

IF YOU LIKE...
Cabernet Sauvignon, Try...
Malbec
Like cab and merlot, malbec is a traditional red Bordeaux blending grape. Today, malbec is the pride of Argentina. These are powerful wines with lots of black fruit. Perfect with steak.

Cabernet Sauvignon: 3 Ways

Red Bordeaux The most famous names—Châteaux Margaux, Lafite, Latour—make powerful and pricey cabs, while the regions of Médoc, Haut-Médoc, and Graves offer great value.
DRINK THIS! **Château Beaumont Haut-Médoc** *2005; $13*

California Cabernet Widely planted throughout California, with Napa being the King of Cabs. The best Napa wines can age for decades and sell for thousands, while up-and-comer areas, like Paso Robles, offer good values.
DRINK THIS! **J. Lohr Estates Seven Oaks Paso Robles Cabernet Sauvignon** *2007; $17*

Southern Hemisphere Cabernet As with merlot, it pays to look south when bargain hunting for cab. Quality is on the rise, with Chile and Australia offering consistent good values.
DRINK THIS! **Yellow Tail Cabernet Sauvignon** *2008, Australia; $8*

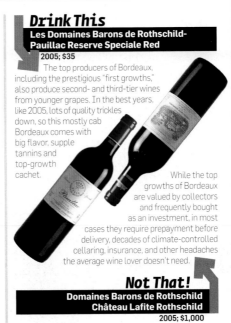

Drink This
Les Domaines Barons de Rothschild-Pauillac Reserve Speciale Red
2005; $35

The top producers of Bordeaux, including the prestigious "first growths," also produce second- and third-tier wines from younger grapes. In the best years, like 2005, lots of quality trickles down, so this mostly cab Bordeaux comes with big flavor, supple tannins and top-growth cachet.

While the top growths of Bordeaux are valued by collectors and frequently bought as an investment, in most cases they require prepayment before delivery, decades of climate-controlled cellaring, insurance, and other headaches the average wine lover doesn't need.

Not That!
Domaines Barons de Rothschild Château Lafite Rothschild
2005; $1,000

Cabernet Sauvignon-Friendly Foods

A simple rule is the bigger the wine, the bigger the food. Add to that cabernet's generous tannins, which help to balance food by bonding with fat and protein, and you have the perfect partner for your boldest flavors.

BEST SNACK
Empanadas

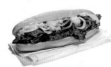

BEST TAKEOUT
Philly cheesesteak

BEST DINNER PARTY
Filet mignon

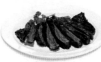

BEST COOKOUT
Flank or skirt steak

Fuel Your Brain

Not only is cabernet sauvignon a thinking man's wine, it might improve your thinking. Researchers at Mount Sinai School of Medicine provided cabernet sauvignon with the drinking water of mice disposed to Alzheimer's disease and determined that it lowered the increased levels of beta-amyloid peptides building up in their brains. These beta-amyloids are a source of neuron-damaging plaque in the brain that can indicate dementia and Alzheimer's disease. Researchers suggest moderate consumption of one drink per day for women and two drinks for men can help reduce the risk of Alzheimer's disease.

Sparkling Wine

● While many Americans are content to fill their day with fizzy cola, for some reason we think sparkling wine is only for wedding toasts and launching ships. While champagne, which comes only from the Champagne region of France, can be quite costly, plenty of affordable alternatives from Spain, Italy, Australia, and the US mean anyone can enjoy a little fizz in their wine. Plus the bubbles and acidity make them some of the most food-friendly and versatile wines around.

AROMA:
Medium to full

BODY
Medium to full

ACIDITY
High

AGING POTENTIAL
None to mid-term (5-10 years)

RESVERATROL
Very low

Segura Viudas Aria Estate Brut
Nonvintage, Spain; $11

Tropical fruit, almond, and honey aromas, but still pleasantly dry.

Argyle Brut
2006, Oregon; $28

Rich with apple, pear, vanilla, and toasty oak flavors.

Nicolas Feuillatte Brut Champagne
Nonvintage, France; $36

Pretty spice, caramelized peaches, and hints of roasted nuts.

IF YOU LIKE...

Sparkling Wine, Try . . .
Sparkling Saké
If you like beer and champy, why not sparkling saké? Serve it chilled, like all bubbly drinks, and take advantage of the touch of sweetness and crisp acidity by pairing with some spicy Asian food.

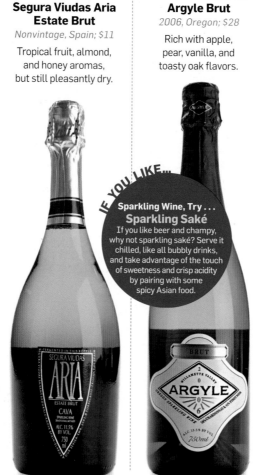

Sparkling Wine: 3 Ways

Champagne The granddaddy of them all, champagne is produced under strict regulations and is usually a blend of chardonnay, pinot noir, and pinot meunier grapes. Expect to pay.

DRINK THIS! Piper-Heidsieck Brut Cuvee *Nonvintage, France; $29*

Cava This sparkling wine comes from approved regions throughout Spain and is fermented in the bottle to create bubbles, just like champagne. However, the grapes are a pure Spanish mouthful: macabeo, parellada, and xarel-lo.

DRINK THIS! Segura Viudas Reserva Heredad *Nonvintage, Spain; $20*

Prosecco Easy to remember, this Italian bubbly is made from the Prosecco grape in the Prosecco region. Because it gets its bubbles by fermenting in a large tank, rather than individual bottles, it's cheaper to make than most bubbly.

DRINK THIS! Mionetto Sergio Brut *Nonvintage, Italy; $16*

Drink This
Veuve Clicquot Brut Champagne
Nonvintage, France; $36

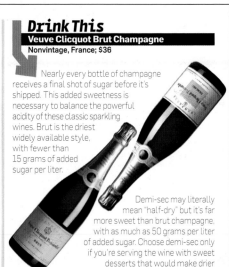

Nearly every bottle of champagne receives a final shot of sugar before it's shipped. This added sweetness is necessary to balance the powerful acidity of these classic sparkling wines. Brut is the driest widely available style, with fewer than 15 grams of added sugar per liter.

Demi-sec may literally mean "half-dry" but it's far more sweet than brut champagne, with as much as 50 grams per liter of added sugar. Choose demi-sec only if you're serving the wine with sweet desserts that would make drier champagne seem too acidic.

Not That!
Veuve Clicquot Demi-Sec Champagne
Nonvintage, France; $45

Sparkling Wine-Friendly Foods
The bubbling action of sparkling wine, combined with bright acidity, make it like a Roomba for your tongue, ready to clean up after fatty, creamy, salty, or lightly spicy foods.

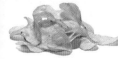

BEST SNACK
Potato chips

BEST TAKEOUT
French fries

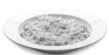

BEST DINNER PARTY
Parmesan risotto

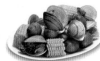

BEST COOKOUT
Clam bake

Drink This, Not That!
Wine Decoder

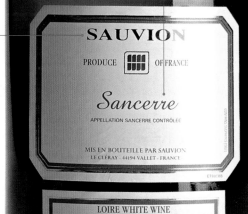

Producer
The person or company that makes the wine, i.e., the brand.

Read a Wine Label

While the FDA has made it easier to find nutrition on food labels, wine labels can still read like heiroglyphics to the untrained eye. The largest type could be the producer, the region, or the grape, depending on which is deemed most important. Here's how to decode a bottle.

Alcohol

Expressed as a percent, alcohol does not directly influence quality. However, it's a good number to be aware of because dry table wines can range from a 10 percent German riesling to a 16 percent California zinfandel. In addition to speeding your buzz, alcohol is the most calorie-intensive part of most wines, with 7 calories per gram, right between a carbohydrate and a fat.

TIP: American wineries can list the alcohol as much as 1.5 percent higher or lower for wine below 14 percent alcohol.

Region

The region is one of the best indications of quality. Each country carefully delineates the boundaries of its quality wine regions. Many Old World regions also dictate details such as the types of grapes, vineyards yields, and ripeness of the fruit. TIP: In both New and Old World wines the region may be vast, or may get as specific as a single vineyard or even a specific block, or section, within a vineyard. Generally speaking, the more specific a wine's region, the higher-priced the wine.

Grape Variety

Wines of the Americas, Australia, and South Africa clearly list the grape variety. These non-European wines are known as New World wines. However, in much of Europe (the Old World), you are expected to know the grape variety that is grown in each region. For instance, white Sancerre isn't the grape, but the region, and whites from this region are made Sauvignon Blanc grapes. TIP: In America, a wine must contain 75 percent of a single grape to list that grape on its label.

Importer

An often-overlooked piece of information, the importer is the person who brings the wine to market. Remember the names of importers of wines that you enjoy and they can help lead you to other wines of comparable taste or quality.

Picking the Perfect Glass

While the fancy crystal manufacturers would have us believe that California merlot won't taste right out of a Right Bank Bordeaux glass, those with limited cabinet space and funds can get a lot of enjoyment from a single versatile glass. Choose your glass based upon its price and its function. The job of a wine glass is to release and concentrate aromas. Therefore, you want a glass that has a bowl large enough to comfortably give the wine a swirl, which increases surface area and releases aromas, and a narrower top, which concentrates these aromas and targets them to your nose. Our favorite glass is the Festival Bordeaux made by Spiegelau, which will cost you about $15 for two glasses (www.glassware.riedel.com).

Drink This, Not That!
Wine 101

Not-So-Pearly Whites

If you choose to drink white wine, do it for the flavor, not to protect your teeth. Researchers at New York University say that drinking white wine also increases the potential for staining your teeth. By soaking cow's teeth in white wine, then exposing the teeth to tea, the researchers determined that teeth are more prone to dark staining following exposure to any wine, whether red or white. While red is still the bigger offender, the acid in white wine also creates rough spots on your teeth, allowing stains to penetrate. A whitening toothpaste is the best defense. On the plus side, researchers have recently learned that components in red wine help battle the bacteria that cause tooth decay.

Widen Your Wine World

While these classic grapes rank far below chardonnay and cabernet in total sales, they are still great grapes to have in your arsenal.

	RIESLING	MALBEC	TEMPRANILLO	SANGIOVESE	NEBBIOLO
FIND IT	Germany; Alsace, France; New York state	Argentina; Cahors, France	Rioja and Ribera del Duero, Spain	Tuscany, Italy; California	Piedmonte, Italy
PAIR IT	Pork, spicy Thai, and Chinese	Grilled meats	Tapas, hard cheeses	Pizza, pasta, and red sauce	Osso bucco and other braised meats
TRY IT	S.A. Prüm Essence Riesling 2008, Mosel, Germany; $12.50	Crios de Susana Balbo Malbec Mendoza 2007, Argentina; $15	Campo Viejo Crianza 2005, Rioja Spain; $9	Castello d'Albola Chianti Classico 2006, Italy; $12	Ceretto 2005 Asij Barbaresco DOCG, Italy; $45
TASTE IT	Juicy apricot, peach, apple, and nectarine with flowers and mineral	Black smoky plums and smooth tannins and spice	Easy drinking with sweet cherry, vanilla, and sometimes leather	Medium-bodied, bright and acidic, with cherries and earthy flavors	Rich with violet flowers, tar, and dark fruit

Five Grapes You Should Experience

If variety really is the spice of life, our wine store shelves could use a little seasoning. The narrow selection of varietal wines most of us enjoy represents only a small portion of the estimated 5,000 wine grape varieties in the world. To be fair, many of them are so obscure they are not even made in commercial quantities. However, it can pay to shop off the beaten path. Lesser-known grapes often offer great values in addition to bringing exciting new flavors to the table.

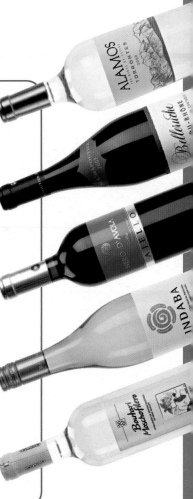

TORRONTES
This aromatic white is grown mainly in Argentina. It's a light, fresh, flowery white that works great with seafood or as an aperitif.

Alamos Torrontes 2009
Argentina; $7

GRENACHE
While this red grape, which goes by garnacha in Spain and cannonau in Italy, gets little respect, it's the second most-planted red in the world. It makes light colored reds with berries and spice and often gets blended with syrah.

M. Chapoutier Côtes-du-Rhône Belleruche Rouge 2007
France; $13

NERO D'AVOLA
Found primarily on the island of Sicily, these reds are rich and dark wines, with rustic fruit, licorice, and peppery flavors along with sweet tannins.

Ajello Nero d'Avola 2007
Sicily; $13

CHENIN BLANC
A native of France's Loire Valley, this white grape is also popular in South Africa, where they make zippy, refreshing wines with aromas of stone fruit, honeysuckle, and pear.

Indaba Chenin Blanc Western Cape 2008
South Africa; $10

MOSCHOFILERO
A Greek white grape with a tongue-twisting name, these wines are highly aromatic with melon, rose petals, and pink grapefruit.

Boutari Moschofilero 2007
Greece; $12

Drink This, Not That!
Wine 202

DRINK TO YOUR HEALTH

Boosting Omega-3s

Omega-3 fatty acids, found in abundance in flax-seed, fish, and olive oil, are believed to help protect against coronary heart disease. A recent study from the Research Laboratories at Catholic University of Campobasso indicates that moderate alcohol consumption, especially of wine consumption, can boost blood levels of omega-3s. Researchers believe that wine acts like a trigger, influencing the metabolism of these essential polyunsaturated fatty acids. Fortunately, several wines pair perfectly with omega-3 rich foods.

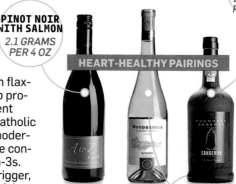

PORT WITH CHEESE AND WALNUTS
2.7 GRAMS PER ¼ CUP

PINOT NOIR WITH SALMON
2.1 GRAMS PER 4 OZ

HEART-HEALTHY PAIRINGS

ZINFANDEL WITH PIZZA DRIZZLED WITH OLIVE OIL
0.2 GRAMS PER OZ

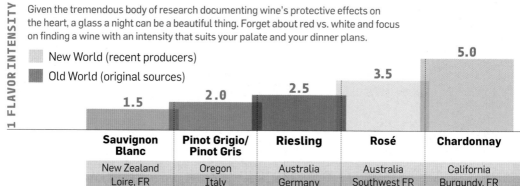

The DTNT Wine Primer

Given the tremendous body of research documenting wine's protective effects on the heart, a glass a night can be a beautiful thing. Forget about red vs. white and focus on finding a wine with an intensity that suits your palate and your dinner plans.

FLAVOR INTENSITY 1 10

☐ New World (recent producers)
☐ Old World (original sources)

	Sauvignon Blanc	Pinot Grigio/ Pinot Gris	Riesling	Rosé	Chardonnay
Intensity	1.5	2.0	2.5	3.5	5.0
New World	New Zealand	Oregon	Australia	Australia	California
Old World	Loire, FR	Italy	Germany	Southwest FR	Burgundy, FR

White, Red, or Green?

How to determine whether your wine is truly eco-friendly

Sustainably Grown

Indicates the grapes come from vineyards that choose natural methods of weed and insect control rather than chemicals.

Certified Organic

Indicates the wine has 95 percent organically grown ingredients with no added sulfites and is monitored throughout its production. The wine may have natural sulfites in fewer than 100 parts per million, while wines that bear the label "made with organic grapes" may carry up to 10 times that amount.

100 Percent Organic

A step above certified organic, these wines use entirely organically certified ingredients and have the same sulfite requirement.

Made from Organically Grown Grapes

These wines are made with a minimum of 70 percent organic ingredients and may have added sulfites. Many organic-ingredient wines fall into this category because winemakers favor using sulfites to make clean tasting and stable wines.

Biodynamic

In addition to being organic, biodynamic grapes are farmed according to the principles of Austrian philosopher Rudolf Steiner. Grapes are planted with attention to planetary cycles and using special soil made from herbs, animals, and minerals.

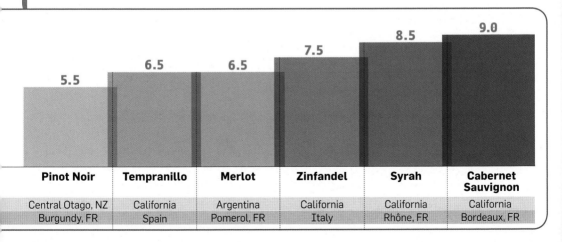

Pinot Noir	Tempranillo	Merlot	Zinfandel	Syrah	Cabernet Sauvignon
5.5	6.5	6.5	7.5	8.5	9.0
Central Otago, NZ Burgundy, FR	California Spain	Argentina Pomerol, FR	California Italy	California Rhône, FR	California Bordeaux, FR

Chapter

9

Drink This, Not That!

BEER & COCKTAILS

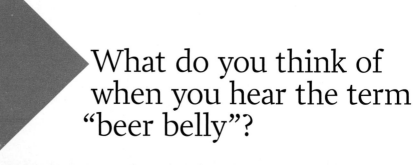

What do you think of when you hear the term "beer belly"?

You might imagine a fat man in a tiny swimsuit, striding across the beach like MacArthur surveying the Pacific Theater, his enormous belly riding above said swimsuit like a ball of dung atop a tiny beetle. Or you think of the guy in the local tavern whose arms have to remain fully extended at all times because his gut is too big to let him "belly up" to the bar.

This is the classic "beer belly"—a round, hard, medicine-ball–style gut that enters the room half a second before its owner. But here's the weird thing: Beer doesn't cause beer bellies.

In fact, drinking beer can help protect against them.

You've probably heard that a drink or two a day has some substantial health effects. For example, beer is rich in silicon, a mineral that plays a key role in increasing bone density. (Not to be confused with silicone, which plays a key role in increasing Kim Kardashian's media exposure.) And the hops used to make beer contain a compound called xanthohumol, which may help protect against some forms of cancer. Moderate drinking has even been linked to lower levels of dementia and heart disease.

But a glass of beer or an occasional cocktail can have yet another, unexpected effect: weight loss!

It's true: In a recent study of more than 8,000 people, Texas Tech University researchers determined that those who downed a daily drink were 54 percent less likely to have a weight problem than teetotalers. Two drinks a day resulted in a 41 percent risk reduction.

But hold on a moment there, Mel Gibson: Two drinks a day is where the trend ends—the minute you ask the bartender to hit you one more time, your risk of obesity starts to climb.

For the moderate drinker, it's not the occasional lager or vodka that will add two fingers to your waistline—it's all the accoutrements, from bar foods to mixers. See, your body sees alcohol as a toxin—which, of course, it is. When you drink, your body goes into overtime trying to burn it off quickly. That means whatever you ingest—the wings, the bar nuts, that scary margarita mix with the nuclear glow—gets secondary treatment. So those calories are more likely to be stored as fat.

The key, then, is knowing which beers and which mixers will give you the health benefits without the extra pounds. That's the key to a long, happy life—and it will ensure that the next time you stroll along the beach, Greenpeace volunteers won't come along and try to roll you back into the ocean.

Ultimate Guide to Beer

Everything you need to know about the suds you love

The first thing you need to understand about beer is that all breeds fall into one of two categories: lagers or ales. At the brewing level, that's primarily a distinction of fungus. It's the fungus—or more specifically, the yeast—that creates the alcohol and shapes the profile of the brew. For ales, brewers use a bottom-fermenting strain of yeast, and they let it do its work under relatively warm conditions. Lagers, the lighter of the two, rely on top-fermenting yeast and colder temperatures. And how do the differences play out on the tongue? Brewers describe ales as smooth, complex, and sometimes creamy, while lagers garner adjectives such as crisp, clean, and bright.

But that's just the introductory course. Within those two beer categories are literally dozens, maybe hundreds, of beer varietals encompassing every shade of tan, copper, brown, and black. There are niche beers infused with herbs and fruit; cider beers; and barley wine (actually beer despite the name). Beer can be filtered or unfiltered, a distinction of whether yeast remains behind in the brew. Then of course, there's that whole esoteric world of European beers—weizenbocks, witbiers, altbiers, dunkelweizens, tripels, dubbels, and so on. It would take a lifetime of hangovers to get them all straight. So to prevent you some of the trouble (or perhaps to get you started), we've handpicked the eight groups of suds you're most likely to encounter. It might not amount to a PhD in brewskiology, but it's more than enough to impress your bartender.

American Lager

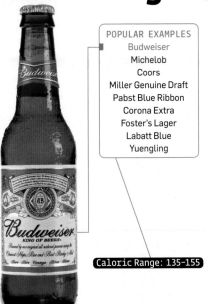

POPULAR EXAMPLES
Budweiser
Michelob
Coors
Miller Genuine Draft
Pabst Blue Ribbon
Corona Extra
Foster's Lager
Labatt Blue
Yuengling

Caloric Range: 135–155

Chances are this is the class of beer you're most familiar with. The biggest producers of American lagers, MillerCoors and Anheuser-Busch InBev, collectively control close to 80 percent of the domestic market. Of all beers, these are the lightest in color and most heavily carbonated. Their closest relatives are the pilsners, but unlike pilsners, which rely solely on barley and hops, these recipes veer toward rice and corn, crops that add little flavor but keep costs low. Plus, a true pilsner is more bitter, with somewhere between 25 and 45 International Units of Bitterness (IBUs). American lagers, with scores as low as 8, are clearly more mellow.

Light Lager

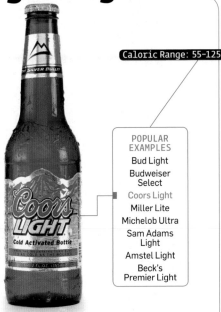

Caloric Range: 55–125

POPULAR EXAMPLES
Bud Light
Budweiser Select
Coors Light
Miller Lite
Michelob Ultra
Sam Adams Light
Amstel Light
Beck's Premier Light

In terms of flavor, these beers aim to replicate American lagers, but they adapt the formula with two key modifications: less alcohol and fewer carbohydrates. Whereas a typical American lager has about 5 percent alcohol, light lagers typically fall between 2.5 and 4.2 percent. And compared with the 8 to 15 grams of carbs in the average American lager, a light lager normally has anywhere between 2 and 9 grams. That makes them your best option for cutting calories. Of course, like American lagers, they lack the complexity of other beer styles. In fact, with the lightest loads of hops and barley, these are considered the least flavorful of all the beers.

Pilsner

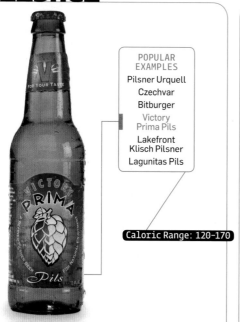

POPULAR
EXAMPLES
Pilsner Urquell
Czechvar
Bitburger
Victory
Prima Pils
Lakefront
Klisch Pilsner
Lagunitas Pils

Caloric Range: 120-170

This is the beer that influences the brewing recipes of American lagers, so if you like the core domestic beers like Bud and Coors, you'll probably love the proper pilsners. Born in the Czech Republic city of Pilsen, these beers are pale, light, and crisp. It's a profile they earn through a simple recipe that relies on four primary ingredients: barley, hops, water, and yeast. (By comparison, Budweiser adds less-flavorful rice to create its brew.) Pilsners, like the American lagers, are tan and gold in color, but they tend to have slightly heavier bodies and less carbonation. Authentic pilsners are difficult to come by in the US. Look to your local microbrew or imports from Europe.

Wheat Beer

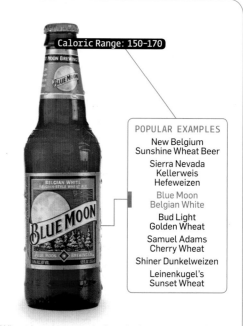

Caloric Range: 150-170

POPULAR EXAMPLES
New Belgium
Sunshine Wheat Beer
Sierra Nevada
Kellerweis
Hefeweizen
Blue Moon
Belgian White
Bud Light
Golden Wheat
Samuel Adams
Cherry Wheat
Shiner Dunkelweizen
Leinenkugel's
Sunset Wheat

Wheat beer is created when the brew master thins out the barley with a significant dose of wheat during the fermentation process. In the US, there are a handful of microbrewers experimenting with wheat lagers. Not in Germany, though. The traditional German wheat beers are always produced as ales, and you'll recognize them by the words "weiss" or "weizen" on the label: weissbier, dunkelweizen, weizenbock, and so on. Compared with barley, wheat carries a heavier load of protein, which plays out as a thicker head in your mug. That protein—along with the fact that many wheat beers are served unfiltered —also helps create the distinctive cloudy look.

Pale Ale

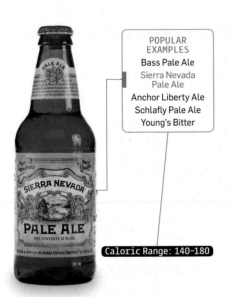

POPULAR EXAMPLES

Bass Pale Ale

Sierra Nevada Pale Ale

Anchor Liberty Ale

Schlafly Pale Ale

Young's Bitter

Caloric Range: 140–180

The American pale ale is predated by the English bitter beers, but today some of the world's best versions are coming from domestic microbreweries. Thankfully these are becoming easier to find. Craft beer sales spiked by 12.4 percent in 2009, and now capture nearly 6 percent of the beer market. It's still in the niche category, but it's a niche with enough support that you shouldn't have trouble digging up a local brew. Although to a lesser degree than in a lager, pale ales are crisp and carbonated, but with the bitterness of pilsner. Amber ale is a close relative; it's just a couple shades darker and leaves a stronger caramel impression on your taste buds.

IPA

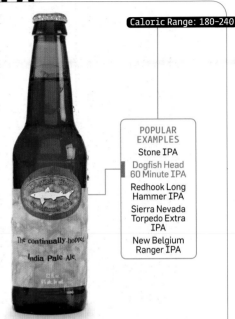

Caloric Range: 180–240

POPULAR EXAMPLES

Stone IPA

Dogfish Head 60 Minute IPA

Redhook Long Hammer IPA

Sierra Nevada Torpedo Extra IPA

New Belgium Ranger IPA

Looking for an ale with a little more oomph? This could be your beer. IPAs, or India pale ales, bring in loads of hops to cut through the sweetness of the barley, often leaving a lingering bitter taste on the tongue. The strongest variety—both in terms of bitterness and alcohol—is the imperial IPA, an ultra-heady brew that cranks the hop levels to maximum. Despite being high in calories, hop-heavy beers have advantages. Researchers at Jerusalem's Hebrew University found that IPAs were significant sources of polyphenols, a class of antioxidants that can lower your cholesterol and decrease your risk of cancer. Now you can officially drink to your health.

Porter

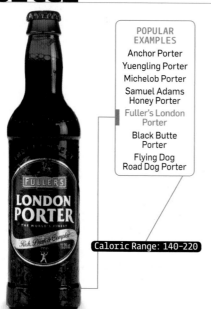

Caloric Range: 140–220

These beers aren't quite as dark as stouts, but they generally fall outside the brown-colored beer spectrum. Of course, you might still sometimes find a light-colored porter sold as a "brown porter." With beers this dark, the lines sometimes blur, but they are defined by strong barley flavors with mild hops. The key to both color and flavor is in the roast of the barley; craft beers generally are blends of brown, chocolate, and black malts. This can play out on your palate like toffee and roasted nuts or sweet licorice and toast. These are medium- to full-bodied beers that go down thick and smooth. Think chocolate milk.

Stout

Caloric Range: 125–230

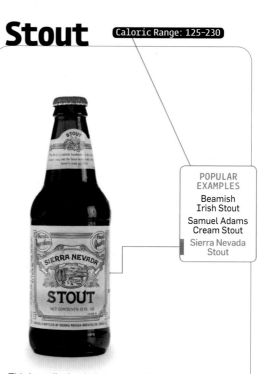

This is easily the darkest breed of beer, often pushing toward completely black. Like porters, stouts pull much of their flavor from the sugars in roasted barley, but they balance this with a slightly heavier reliance on bitter hops. Casual drinkers are some-times put off by the color, but generally these beers are very palatable. They're creamy with undertones of coffee and chocolate, and many of them are served with slightly less alcohol than the average full-bodied beer. Guinness Draught, for instance, delivers only 4 percent alcohol. But be warned: Those labeled "extra stout" are a stronger breed and often carry alcohol loads as high as 8 percent.

Beer, Meet Food

Food and wine have always had a symbiotic relationship; chefs and sommeliers alike use one to enhance the other, turning to an intense merlot to bolster the beefiness of a ribeye or a crisp sauvignon blanc to match the subtle sweetness of a fillet of sole. But beer and food? Absolutely, says a chorus of America's best chefs and brewmasters. "Good food can make good beer taste better, and vice versa," says Aviram Turgeman, a beer sommelier at Cafe D'Alsace in Manhattan. Here's how he matches the two.

FOOD/BEER	WHY IT WORKS	HEALTH BONUS	PERFECT PICK
Food **Pizza, Mackerel** **Beer** **Pilsner, Lager**	**Structure.** A dry, crisp beer with balanced hops can overcome strong flavors such as the seasonings on a pizza or the oiliness of fish. Plus, hops scrub your tastebuds between bites.	When steak was soaked in pilsner for 6 hours before cooking, a carcinogen in the meat was reduced by as much as 88 percent, according to a recent study.	**Jever Pilsener** *Also try...* Stella Artois, Kronenbourg 1664
Food **Burger, Chicken, Lamb** **Beer** **Amber Ale**	**Intensity.** "Strong flavors overwhelm light beers," says Turgeman. That's why you need a complex, heavier brew to handle this hearty fare.	A 2007 study found that the hops in a beer like an amber ale may help lower cholesterol and prevent blood clotting.	**Fischer Amber** *Also try...* Sierra Nevada Pale Ale, Samuel Smith's Nut Brown Ale
Food **Sausage, Roast Pork** **Beer** **Farmhouse Ale**	**Region.** European beers + European food = great paring. Carry the lesson to other cuisines, to complement undertones in each: Asian beer with sushi, a Mexican cerveza with tacos, and so on.	The barley used in ale's brewing process contains flavonoids, a group of compounds that may interfere with the multiplication of cancer cells.	**Saison Dupont** *Also try...* La Choulette Blonde, Castelain Blond
Food **Green Salad, Egg** **Beer** **Belgian White**	**Weight/body.** Citrus-packed, lighter wheat beers make food taste fresher and cut through the richness of yolks or hollandaise sauce.	Compounds in wheat beers may help lower your risk of cardiovascular diseases, say Austrian researchers.	**Gruut Belgian Wit Beer** *Also try...* Hoegaarden, Blue Moon
Food **Cheese, Salmon** **Beer** **Trappist, Abbey**	**Body/strength.** The mild sweetness and yeastiness of Trappist beers play off the charred flavors of smoked or grilled food or pungent cheese.	Brewer's yeast contains B vitamins, protein, and minerals, but it rests on the bottom in Trappist beer bottles. So pour your beer into a glass and swirl.	**Chimay Red** *Also try...* Leffe Blonde, Goose Island Matilda
Food **Chocolate, Fruit** **Beer** **Stout, Porter, Flavored Lambics**	**There are no rules.** "Experiment with sweet beers," Turgeman says. "You can make great combinations." To cap off a dinner date, pair chocolate with cherry lambic.	The black-cherry juice in cherry lambics is higher in disease-fighting antioxidants than cranberry and orange juice are, a 2008 UCLA study found.	**Lindemans Kriek Lambic** *Also try...* Smuttynose Robust Porter, Young's Double Chocolate Stout

Drink This, Not That!

Get a Handle on the Hard Stuff

Everything you need to know about liquor

Believe it or not, there are benefits to drinking booze. Numerous large surveys have come to the conclusion that much of the same benefits derived from red wine can also be found with a slug of vodka or a snifter of brandy. In small amounts, ethanol, the pure form of alcohol found in beer, wine, and spirits, has been shown to raise HDL ("good") cholesterol, encourage better blood flow, and increase insulin sensitivity.

Nowhere is ethanol more concentrated than on the liquor shelf, where the main spirits contain anywhere from 35 to 60 percent pure alcohol. But with greater strength comes greater risk. A light cocktail may deliver some

of the same benefits as a glass of pinot, but a barrage of Jäger shots—or even an extra large martini—will do the exact opposite, increasing your risk for cardiovascular disease and an early death. Talk about a buzz kill.

Don't fret. You can have your whisky and drink it, too, just as long as you understand the difference between sipping for enjoyment and slurping for sheer intoxication. It helps to start by equipping yourself with a solid understanding of the variety of white and brown liquors out there—how they're made, how they taste, and how strong of a punch they pack. It's all in the name of making you a smarter— and safer—drinker.

Vodka

Rum

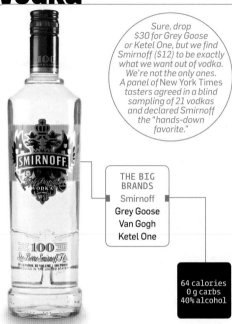

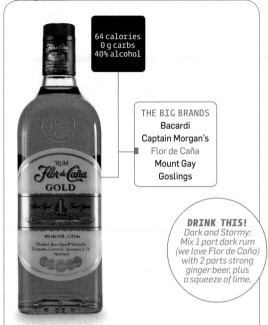

Sure, drop $30 for Grey Goose or Ketel One, but we find Smirnoff ($12) to be exactly what we want out of vodka. We're not the only ones. A panel of New York Times tasters agreed in a blind sampling of 21 vodkas and declared Smirnoff the "hands-down favorite."

64 calories
0 g carbs
40% alcohol

THE BIG BRANDS
Bacardi
Captain Morgan's
Flor de Caña
Mount Gay
Goslings

THE BIG BRANDS
Smirnoff
Grey Goose
Van Gogh
Ketel One

64 calories
0 g carbs
40% alcohol

DRINK THIS!
Dark and Stormy: Mix 1 part dark rum (we love Flor de Caña) with 2 parts strong ginger beer, plus a squeeze of lime.

America's hooch of choice? Definitely vodka. It drives 28 percent of the liquor market, according to the Distilled Spirits Council. Much of our affinity for vodka stems from the fact that it's the least pronounced of all the liquors, meaning it's more or less a blank canvas for cocktail creation. Generally, vodka production begins by allowing fermentation to create ethanol through the breakdown of starches in wheat, rye, and sometimes potatoes. The ethanol is then distilled, or boiled out from the mix, and heavily filtered to remove any unwanted flavor compounds. That helps it blend unnoticed into drinks such as Bloody Marys, screwdrivers, and apple martinis.

Rum is distilled from either molasses or cane sugar, which makes it a natural choice for daiquiris and piña coladas (and which makes rum-based cocktails among the most consistently high-calorie at the bar). The different shades of rum spring from variations in processing. Fresh-distilled rum is clear, but gold varieties, such as Captain Morgan, have been aged in wooden casks. Clear varieties, like Bacardi Silver, have spent their resting days in tanks of stainless steel. To make dark rum, producers take the wood-barreled rum and flavor it with a few shots of caramel or molasses, which makes it somewhat of a hybrid between liquor and liqueur.

(Nutritional info is for 1 ounce)

Tequila

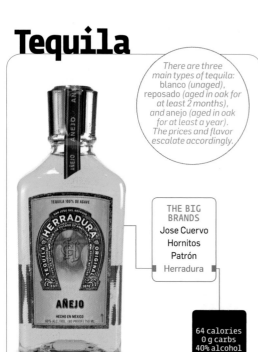

There are three main types of tequila: blanco (unaged), reposado (aged in oak for at least 2 months), and anejo (aged in oak for at least a year). The prices and flavor escalate accordingly.

THE BIG BRANDS
Jose Cuervo
Hornitos
Patrón
Herradura

64 calories
0 g carbs
40% alcohol

From the Mexican agave tequilana, we get tequila. The plant, also called blue agave, is native to the Mexican state Jalisco, and by Mexican law, only those spirits flowing from certain parts of this region can be rightfully called tequila. The purest versions rely solely on the alcohol produced from blue agave, and they're labeled with some variation of the claim "100 percent blue agave." Other varieties, called *mixtos*, pull about half their flavor from agave and half from the fermentation of other cheap sugars such as cane juice. Notice how Jose Cuervo Gold makes no claim about the amount of agave in its bottle? That's a sure-fire sign of mixto.

Gin

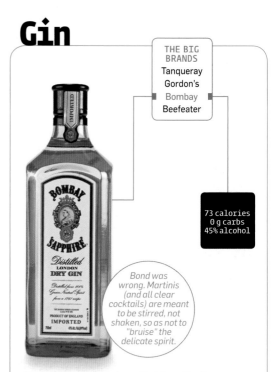

THE BIG BRANDS
Tanqueray
Gordon's
Bombay
Beefeater

73 calories
0 g carbs
45% alcohol

Bond was wrong. Martinis (and all clear cocktails) are meant to be stirred, not shaken, so as not to "bruise" the delicate spirit.

Much like vodka, gin is crafted from the flavor-neutral starches of cereal grains. What makes a gin a gin, however, is the juniper added during distillation. These green-and-blue seed cones, often referred to as berries, impart a tart flavor and create a clean, piney foundation for martinis and gimlets. Studies have also shown them to reduce blood glucose levels in rats. Whereas the best vodkas are smooth and straightforward, the great gins tend to carry complex floral notes and rich bouquets of herbs and spice. Beware though, as major gin producers—Beefeater, Tanqueray—bottle versions slightly above the 80-proof ceiling observed by most spirits.

(Nutritional info is for 1 ounce)

Whiskey

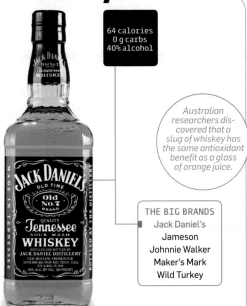

64 calories
0 g carbs
40% alcohol

Australian researchers discovered that a slug of whiskey has the same antioxidant benefit as a glass of orange juice.

THE BIG BRANDS
Jack Daniel's
Jameson
Johnnie Walker
Maker's Mark
Wild Turkey

The flavor of whiskey is subject to a host of nuanced production techniques. Most are made with malted grains, but bourbon—a distinct class of American whiskey—contains at least 51 percent corn. Some varieties, such as most Scotch whiskies (produced, of course, in Scotland), are distilled three times and then all are dumped into barrels for aging, which can take a decade or longer. The type of wood used to make the storage barrels, the length of aging, and the processes of filtering and distilling all contribute to the range of character in the whiskey. Single-malt is often blended back with cheaper grain whiskies to control flavors and lower production costs.

Brandy

The world's most expensive bottle of liquor is a gold- and diamond-encrusted bottle of 100-year-old brandy that sells for $2 million.

THE BIG BRANDS
Hennessey
Rémy Martin
Courvoisier

70 calories
0 g carbs
43% alcohol

Whereas most common liquors are made from grains, the standard brandy owes its distinct flavor to grapes. When fermentation occurs in grapes, we get wine, and when producers distill that wine to filter out the alcohol, we get brandy. Of course, other fruits such as plums, cherries, and apples can be used as well. But among the better-known varieties —cognac, Armagnac, grappa, and so on—grapes are a must. By the time brandy makes it to the liquor store, it has sometimes, but not always, been aged in barrels, and there's a good chance that it's been blended to incorporate the different flavors created by different aging techniques and grape varieties.

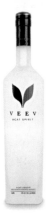

Healthier Hooch?

Savvy distillers are beginning to impart their spirits with antioxidant-rich doses of fruits, spices, and herbs. Is this just clever marketing, or do these newfangled bottles deserve a space on your liquor cabinet?

Veev Acai Spirit

Looks like the South American acai berry has made the leap from smoothie to spirit. That's not such a bad thing, considering that it's one of the most antioxidant-rich foods on the planet.
To complement the Brazilian berry, Veev has also imbued this bottle with shots of prickly pear and acerola cherry as well. And all that fruit is a good sign for cocktail lovers: The USDA found that adding alcohol to fruit increases the fruit's antioxidant capacity. Mix with fresh smashed blackberries, mint, and a splash of soda.

No nutritional information available
30% alcohol

Zen Green Tea

The makers of Zen are trying to combine teatime with happy hour by infusing neutral grain spirits with Japanese tea leaves, lemongrass, and other herbs. It's a good pairing, too; a study published in the journal *Biological Chemistry* showed that green tea protected the liver from some of the oxidative stress brought on by alcohol. Try mixing it with rum in your next mojito, or to stick with the flavor theme, brew up some green tea, ice it down, and pour in a shot.

103 calories
11 carbohydrates
20% alcohol

Pama Pomegranate Liqueur

The crimson tide of pomegranate has already flooded every part of the American supermarket, so why not the liquor store as well? Plenty of research has gone into these vaunted purple orbs, with studies finding them effective in the fight against both prostate and lung cancers. Of course, that dose of defense will always be more concentrated in the fruit itself, but subbing a bit of the liqueur for a normal spirit is a solid swap to make. Try making our Classic Margarita recipe on page 43 with half tequila, half Pama.

85 calories
11 g carbohydrates
17% alcohol

Loft Organic Spicy Ginger

The organic liquor market took off years ago, but eco-friendly liqueurs have been slow to emerge. Loft was the first of its kind to be certified USDA organic, and even now its distribution is limited to the West Coast and New York. But with flavors like lemongrass, blueberry, and tangerine, it's only a matter of time before it moves inland. The spirits are shot through with organic fruits and herbs, with only enough refined sugar to meet the legal definition of a liqueur. The real sugar hit comes from organic agave nectar, a gentler source of sweetness. Find a distributor at LoftLiqueurs.com.

No nutritional information available
25% alcohol

Bottom Line

These lines of liqueurs aren't going to cure cancer or magically shrink your waistline, but they will up the nutritional ante in your next cocktail ever so slightly. Be warned, though: These all have high sugar contents, so think twice before adding any more sweetness to the mix. Soda water and fresh lime are your best bets.

The Role Players

With strong flavors and even stronger sugar concentrations, these spirits are best sipped sparingly

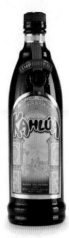

Orange Liqueur

Like most liqueurs, this shot of citrus earns its calories from the one-two punch of sugar and alcohol. Indeed, every carbohydrate in this bottle comes from sugar. When making cocktails with orange liqueurs—whether it be a margarita or a boozy punch—remember to hold off on the added sugar.

Per ounce:
95 calories
7.4 g carbohydrates
40% alcohol

THE BIG BRANDS

Grand Marnier

Curaçao

McGuinness Triple Sec

Schnapps

In the traditional German sense, schnapps denotes a brandy-like liquor that was distilled from fermented fruit and bottled without sugar. But leave it to America to find a cheaper method. The schnapps we drink today is generally no more than grain alcohol swirled with a slough of sweeteners, flavors, and colors. That being said, it does have one nutritional advantage over other liqueurs, and that's the lower alcohol content.

Per ounce:
72 calories
8.1 g carbohydrates
15% alcohol

THE BIG BRANDS

DeKuyper Sour Apple Pucker

99 Blackberries

Archers Peach Schnapps

Bols Butterscotch Schnapps

Herb-and-Spice Liqueur

According to Jäger-meister, there are 56 different ingredients at work in this bottle. The one that stands out, however, is anise, the herb that hits your palate like a lash from a black licorice vine. Indeed, herbal liqueurs are among the most interesting and complex flavors in the liquor store, but when it comes to empty calories, they're just as guilty as every other bottle on the shelf. Be sure to proceed cautiously.

Per ounce:
103 calories
11 g carbohydrates
35% alcohol

THE BIG BRANDS

Jägermeister

Galliano

Goldschlager

Chartreuse

Nut Liqueur

Whether made from almonds, walnuts, or hazelnuts, nut liqueurs tend to share a few things in common: low alcohol content, high sugar concentration, and an Italian heritage. Forget drinks like the amaretto sour (which can pack 300 calories or more) and be judicious when using these potent bottles. Ditch the glass and try a splash over a bowl of vanilla ice cream as an adult alternative to a hot fudge sundae.

Per ounce:
79 calories
11.8 g carbohydrates
21% alcohol

THE BIG BRANDS

Barton's Amaretto Di Amore

Frangelico

Nocello

Bellota

Coffee Liqueur

The jolt you get from a swig of Kahlúa is less likely to be from the alcohol or the caffeine (despite the name, coffee liqueurs tend to be low in each) and more likely to be a side effect of the massive amounts of sugar it contains. If you're going to drink, try diffusing the sweetness in a cup of hot coffee.

Per ounce:
91 calories
14.7 g carbohydrates
20% alcohol

THE BIG BRANDS

Kahlúa

Tia Maria

Starbucks Coffee Liqueur

Patrón XO Cafe

The World's Healthiest

A spoonful of sugar helps the medicine go down, but then so does a shot of organic vodka. That's the philosophy of a crafty crew of mixologists we've gathered from some of the best bars in the country. If you're going for the buzz, you might as well get some benefits, right?

THE BENEFIT: Lutein, which is found in carrots, can reduce your risk of cancer, says an American Journal of Clinical Nutrition *study.*

The Rabbit Hole

3 oz fresh carrot juice
⅓ oz fresh cucumber juice
½ oz Cynar, an Italian herbal liqueur
1 oz organic vodka
1 sprig sage

Combine the liquid ingredients in a shaker with ice. Shake and strain into a cocktail glass. Top with the sage sprig.

From Greg Best, mixologist at Restaurant Eugene, Atlanta, GA

Pepper Delicious

3 red bell pepper slices
6-8 fresh mint leaves
2 oz gin
1 oz fresh lime juice
¾ oz simple syrup
(equal parts sugar and water)

In a shaker glass, combine 2 red pepper rings and the mint leaves and press firmly with a muddler to pulverize the peppers. Add the gin, lime juice, syrup, and ice. Shake and strain into a chilled glass. Garnish with the remaining pepper ring.

From Ryan Magarian, president of Liquid Relations, Portland, OR

THE BENEFIT: A diet high in vitamin C, carotenoids, and lycopene (all of which are amply supplied in red peppers) reduces the incidence of chronic disease and death, according to a Spanish study of 41,000 people.

Cocktails

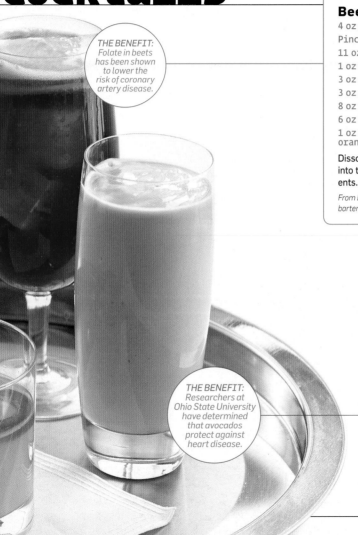

THE BENEFIT:
Folate in beets has been shown to lower the risk of coronary artery disease.

Beet Sangria

4 oz sugar
Pinch of salt
11 oz beet juice
1 oz fresh lime juice
3 oz fresh OJ
3 oz ginger beer (or ale)
8 oz red wine
6 oz brandy
1 oz Cointreau or other orange liqueur

Dissolve the sugar and salt into the nonalcoholic ingredients. Add the alcohol and stir.

From Eben Freeman, former bartender at Tailor, New York, NY

THE BENEFIT:
Researchers at Ohio State University have determined that avocados protect against heart disease.

Avocado Daiquiri

4 oz rum (a mix of gold and silver is best)
¼ medium-ripe avocado
½ oz half-and-half
¼ oz fresh lemon or lime juice
2 oz simple syrup (equal parts sugar and water)
1⅓ cups ice cubes

Combine the ingredients and blend until smooth.

From Hip Sips, *by Lucy Brennan*

Drink This

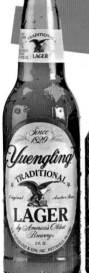

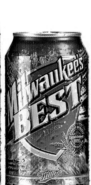

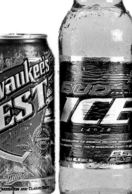

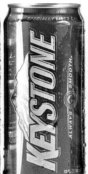

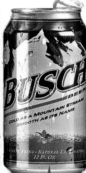

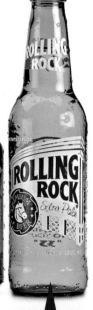

Yuengling Lager

135 calories
12 g carbs
4.4% alcohol

America's oldest brewery makes a basic lager that trumps most full-flavored beers in terms of calories.

Milwaukee's Best

128 calories
11.4 g carbs
4.3% alcohol

"The Beast" and all its spin-offs are on the lighter side of the caloric spectrum.

Bud Ice

123 calories
3.8 g carbs
5.5% alcohol

By keeping the carbs in check, Bud Ice manages to make itself the most alcohol-heavy beer at fewer than 125 calories a bottle.

Keystone Premium

111 calories
5.8 g carbs
4.43% alcohol

Choose Keystone Premium over Keystone Light and you'll suffer a mere 6 extra calories per can.

Busch

133 calories
10.2 g carbs
4.6% alcohol

Anheuser's economy beer trumps both Budweiser and Michelob, the company's two more prominent lines.

Rolling Rock Extra Pale

132 calories
10 g carbs
4.5% alcohol

One of the few low-calorie beers with a real flavor profile. Pair with shrimp cocktail for a killer low-calorie combo.

The kings of domestic beers tend to be lagers and pilsners, two relatively light styles of beers. Look to get your fix for under 140 calories a bottle—and hopefully much lower.

Not That!

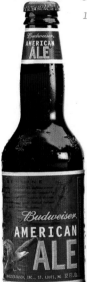

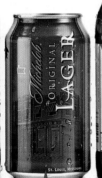

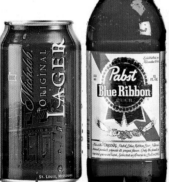

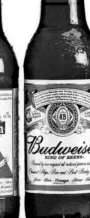

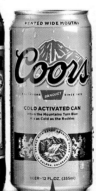

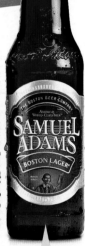

Budweiser American Ale

182 calories
18.1 g carbs
3.2% alcohol

The worst of Bud's mainstream bottles.

Michelob

155 calories
13.3 g carbs
5% alcohol

If you're going the Michelob route, make sure it's Michelob Ultra.

Pabst Blue Ribbon

144 calories
12.8 g carbs
5% alcohol

PBR may be experiencing a revival in hipster circles, but it's still an average beer at best.

Budweiser

144 calories
12.8 g carbs
4.7% alcohol

The self-proclaimed King of Beers has been usurped by his icy brother.

Coors Banquet

149 calories
12.2 g carbs
5% alcohol

Apparently tapping the Rockies has only had adverse effects on Coors' calorie counts.

Samuel Adams Boston Lager

170 calories
18 g carbs
4.9% alcohol

Sam Adams makes some of the tastiest beers in America. Too bad they're all so high in calories.

303

LIGHT BEER
Drink This

Michelob Ultra Pomegranate Raspberry

107 calories
6 g carbs
4% alcohol

If you must drink flavored beers, this is your best option.

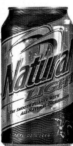

Budweiser's recently released Select 55 is the lowest-calorie beer on the market.

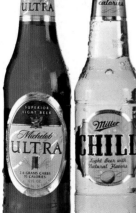
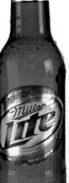
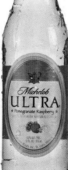
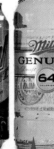
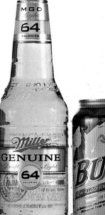
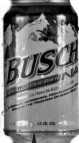

Michelob Ultra

95 calories
2.6 g carbs
4.2% alcohol

Virtually the same amount of alcohol, but with less than a third of the carbs.

Miller Chill

100 calories
4 g carbs
4.2% alcohol

It's identical to Bud Light Lime in every way except that it's 16 calories lighter. Not a huge savings, but are you really in a position to throw away calories?

Miller Lite

96 calories
3.2 g carbs
4.2% alcohol

Miller makes some of the most reliable low-carb, low-cal beers on the market.

Natural Light

95 calories
3.2 g carbs
4.2% alcohol

Nearly identical nutritionally to Michelob Ultra, which puts it in good company.

MGD 64

64 calories
2.4 g carbs
2.8% alcohol

This is the lightest beer you can purchase under the Miller logo, and the second lightest under any logo.

Busch NA

60 calories
12.9 g carbs
0.4% alcohol

"Nonalcoholic" beer is made like any other beer, only the alcohol is removed after the brewing.

Not That!

Bud Light & Clamato Chelada

151 calories
15.6 g carbs
4.2% alcohol

Clamato is loaded with high-fructose corn syrup and MSG. No thanks!

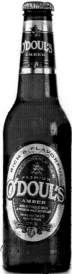
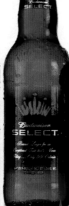
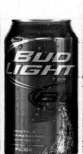
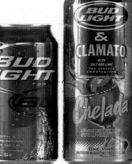

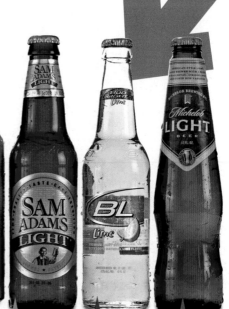

O'Doul's Amber

90 calories
18 g carbs
0.4% alcohol

They may have cut the alcohol, but they sure didn't skimp on the carbs.

Budweiser Select

99 calories
3.1 g carbs
4.3% alcohol

A decent beer by any standard, but if you're really trying to cut calories, 64 is the new standard.

Bud Light

110 calories
6.6 g carbs
4.2% alcohol

If you're going light, then your beer shouldn't have more than 100 calories.

Samuel Adams Light

119 calories
9.7 g carbs
4.05% alcohol

It's not the lightest beer on tap, but it is the lightest of Sam's brews by 40 calories.

Bud Light Lime

116 calories
8 g carbs
4.2% alcohol

We give Bud credit for not using the lime flavoring as an excuse to jack the calories. Still, you can do better.

Michelob Light

123 calories
8.8 g carbs
4.3% alcohol

For 2 extra calories you could be drinking a Guinness.

Drink This

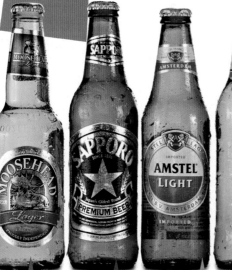
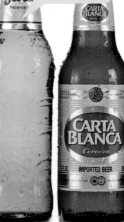
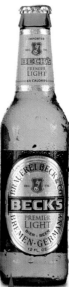
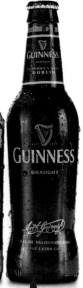

Grolsch Premium Lager

147 calories
10.4 g carbs
5% alcohol

Much better than its Dutch counterpart, Heineken.

Moosehead Pale Ale

135 calories
10.2 carbs
5% alcohol

Moosehead is one of the only large, 100% Canadian-owned breweries left.

Sapporo

140 calories
10.3 g carbs
4.9% alcohol

The best of the major Japanese imports.

Amstel Light

95 calories
5 g carbs
3.5% alcohol

One of our all-time favorite beers. Few beers can claim a better taste-to-calories ratio.

Carta Blanca

128 calories
11 g carbs
4% alcohol

Mexico began producing Carta Blanca in 1890, nearly four decades before the first batch of Corona.

Beck's Premier Light

64 calories
4 g carbs
3.9% alcohol

The lightest import on the market.

Guinness Draught

125 calories
10 g carbs
4% alcohol

Look all you want, but you won't find a darker beer with fewer calories.

With increasing access to high-quality imports, don't settle for a beer short on flavor and long on calories.

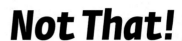

Not That!

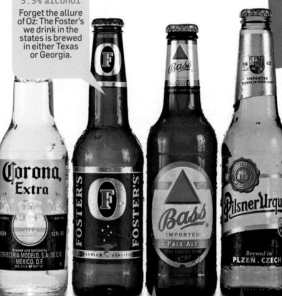

Foster's Premium Ale

160 calories
12.5 g carbs
5.5% alcohol

Forget the allure of Oz: The Foster's we drink in the states is brewed in either Texas or Georgia.

Guinness Extra Stout

176 calories
14 g carbs
6% alcohol

Just make sure you buy the right Guinness. It's a mistake that will cost you 300 calories a six-pack.

Molson Canadian Light

113 calories
9.9 g carbs
3.9% alcohol

Not particularly impressive when compared to other light beers.

Corona Extra

148 calories
14 g carbs
4.6% alcohol

Clear bottles let in more sunlight than brown bottles, and sunlight is the enemy of fresh beer.

Bass

160 calories
13 g carbs
5.5% alcohol

Substitute Amstel for the Bass in a traditional black and tan and you'll make a lighter version with only 110 calories per 12 ounces.

Pilsner Urquell

156 calories
16 g carbs
4.4% alcohol

The national beer of the Czech Replublic suffers from a carb overload.

Heineken

166 calories
9.8 g carbs
5.4% alcohol

For this many calories, we'd expect a more flavorful beer.

CRAFT & MICRO BREWS

Drink This

The American microbrew industry is flourishing, with more small craft brewers opening their doors every day.

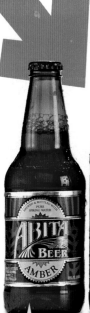
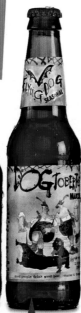
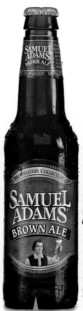
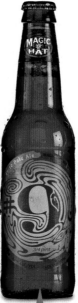
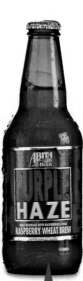
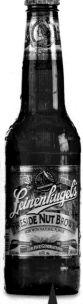

Abita Amber

128 calories
10 g carbs
4.5% alcohol

Perfect for spicy or Cajun food—fitting, as it's brewed in the heart of Creole country.

Flying Dog Dog-toberfest

146 calories
11.4 g carbs
5.3% alcohol

This was the winning German-style Marzen at the 2009 Great American Beer Festival in Denver.

Samuel Adams Brown Ale

160 calories
18 g carbs
5.35% alcohol

Brown ales tend to carry a potent caloric punch. This is as light as it gets, and one of Sam's best beers.

Magic Hat #9

153 calories
14.2 g carbs
5.1% alcohol

This small Vermont Brewery makes big-flavored beers. This is their flagship brew, what they describe as "not quite a pale ale."

Abita Purple Haze

128 calories
11 g carbs
4.2% alcohol

A wheat beer tinged with raspberry puree added at the end of the brewing process. Try it with a hunk of brie on the side.

Leinenkugel's Fireside Nut Brown

155 calories
13.4 g carbs
4.9% alcohol

Dark craft beers tend to tow an extra load of carbs behind all that flavor.

Not That!

Craft beers tend to be long on alcohol and carbs, which means finding a beer with fewer than 150 calories becomes a real challenge. We do our best to assist.

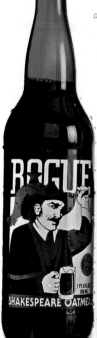
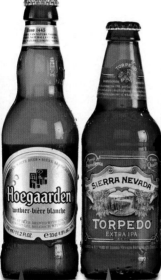
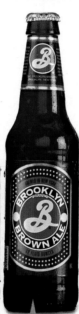
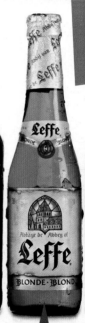
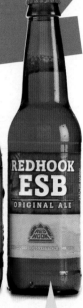

Rogue Brewery Shakespeare Oatmeal Stout
(per 12 fl oz)

201 calories
13.2 g carbs
6% alcohol

The Bard should stick to writing sonnets.

Hoegaarden

176 calories
13 g carbs
4.9% alcohol

One of the oldest beers on the planet, started in Belgium in 1445. Too bad it doesn't have better nutritionals to match all that history.

Sierra Nevada Extra IPA

236 calories
20.6 g carbs
7.2% alcohol

Of the 13 Sierra beers, more than half weigh in at more than 200 calories.

Brooklyn Brown Ale

205 calories
15 g carbs
5.6% alcohol

Brooklyn makes great, increasingly popular beers. What they don't do, though, is make light beers.

Leffe Blonde Beer

200 calories
17 g carbs
6.6% alcohol

Another example of a high-calorie Belgium beer unfit for regular consumption.

Redhook ESB Original Ale

179 calories
14.2 g carbs
5.8% alcohol

This Extra Special Bitter beer packs quite a caloric wallop.

309

Drink This

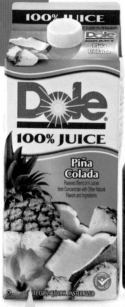

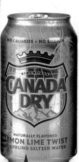

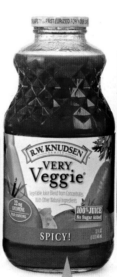

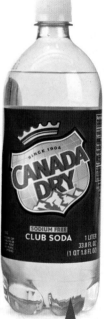

Dole
Piña Colada
(4 fl oz)

60 calories
0 g fat
12.5 g sugars

You'll find this 100% juice blend in the cooler. Mix three parts juice with one part rum and garnish with a hunk of fresh pineapple.

Canada Dry
Lemon Lime
Twist Sparkling
Seltzer Water
(12 fl oz)

0 calories
0 g fat
0 g sugars

Seltzer water is calorie-free, and with the added lemon twist, it's a good as sugar-free 7Up.

R.W. Knudsen
Very Veggie
Spicy!
(8 fl oz)

50 calories
0 g fat
7 g sugars
590 mg sodium

This 100% juice includes tomatoes, jalapenos, and celery—perfect for a Bloody Mary.

Canada Dry
Club Soda
(8 fl oz)

0 calories
0 g fat
0 g sugars

Want something bubbly in your drink to cut the booze? Make it plain soda, the best mixer of all.

Not That!

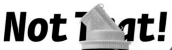

Because all of the major spirits have around the same amount of calories, it's the mixers that make or break your cocktail.

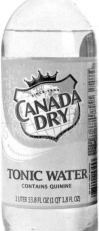

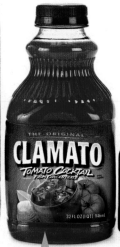

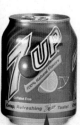

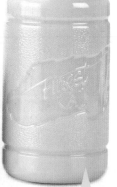

Canada Dry Tonic
(8 fl oz)

90 calories
0 g fat
23 g sugars

Tonic has grown sweeter and sweeter over the years, to the point where it's now nearly indistinguishable from, say, Sprite.

Clamato Tomato Cocktail
(8 fl oz)

60 calories
0 g fat
8 g sugars
880 mg sodium

Clamato is only 35% real juice, and each serving provides a staggering 880 mg sodium. That's a third of your day's intake.

7Up
(8 fl oz)

100 calories
0 g fat
25 g sugars

Soda of any variety makes for a calorie-loaded cocktail. And don't think you'll escape with diet. Researchers in Australia found that diet mixers can intensify the effects of alcohol.

Finest Call Premium Piña Colada Mix
(4 fl oz)

210 calories
1.5 g fat
(1 g saturated)
52 g sugars

Wow, every drink you pour will have as much sugar as 3½ Little Debbie Marshmallow Pies.

Drink This

Premade mixers are the bane of the cocktail world. Most are made primarily of high-fructose corn syrup and artificial colorings. If you want a ready-to-go mixer, look to Stirrings. At least their stuff is made with real juice.

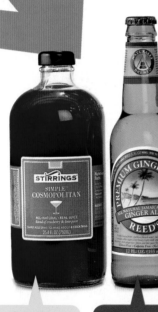
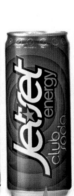
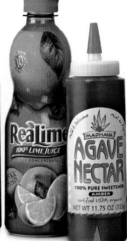
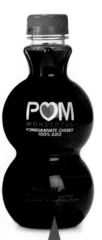

Stirrings Simple Cosmopolitan Mix (3 fl oz)
60 calories
0 g fat
16 g sugar

Made with real cranberry and key lime juices—a rarity in the world of mixers.

Reed's Premium Ginger Brew (8 fl oz)
100 calories
0 g fat
22 g sugars

Ginger beer is made with a larger dose of ginger than ginger ale, which is why we'll cough up the extra 10 calories here.

JetSet Club Soda Energy Mixer (10.5 fl oz can)
0 calories
0 g fat
0 g sugars

Like Red Bull, JetSet's Club Soda is loaded with taurine, caffeine, and B vitamins, just without all the sugar.

3 Tbsp ReaLime 100% Lime Juice and 1 Tbsp Madhava Agave Nectar
50 calories
0 g fat
15 g sugar

This is how real margaritas are made, with fresh lime juice and a hint of sugar.

Pom Wonderful 100% Juice Pomegranate Cherry (4 fl oz)
75 calories
0 g fat
16.5 g sugars

These are natural sugars, which means you get nutrients, too.

Not That!

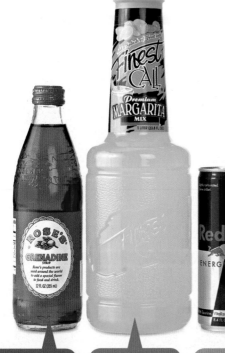
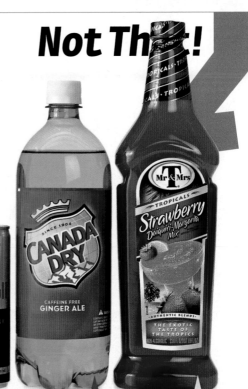

Rose's Grenadine
(2 Tbsp)

90 calories
0 g fat
21 g sugars

Looks fruity. Tastes fruity. Yet in truth, there's not a shred of fruit in this syrupy cocktail staple.

Finest Call Premium Margarita Mix
(4 fl oz)

160 calories
0 g fat
38 g sugars

Real margaritas don't contain corn-based sweeteners or artificial colors. Consider this the crutch of the amateur.

Red Bull
(8.4 fl oz can)

110 calories
0 g fat
27 g sugars

Be cautious when mixing alcohol with energy drinks. Research has shown people drinking both tend to underestimate their levels of intoxication.

Canadian Dry Ginger Ale
(8 fl oz)

90 calories
0 g fat
24 g sugars

Better for you than 7Up or Sprite, since Canadian Dry also contains real ginger. Still, we prefer the stronger stuff.

Mr and Mrs T's Strawberry Daiquiri-Margarita Mix
(4 fl oz)

180 calories
0 g fat
44 g sugars

Mostly high-fructose corn syrup and food coloring— enough to spoil any good drink.

Index

Boldface page references indicate photographs.
<u>Underscored</u> references indicate boxed text.

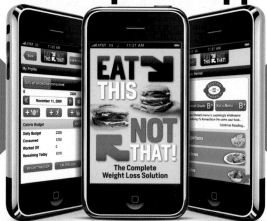